Type 2 Diabetes Wellness Region

Mr Dennis E Lutz

Contents

Notice to readers

This book is written with the express purpose of sharing what the Author has learned about his experience with Type 2 diabetes. and his success in reversing the complications (not curing) for his disease. Consequently, the information in this book is not intended to prescribe any form of treatment for any illness.

The FDA has not verified any claims. To obtain appropriate recommendation to particular situation, please consult a qualified specialist.

Chapter 1
What Is Diabetes

With diabetes such an epidemic today, it is essential that you know exactly what it is. Why? Well, to prevent getting diabetes yourself that is! In layman terms, "diabetes" is the inability of the body to process sugars properly. When we eat or drink, our "pancreas" produces a hormone called "insulin". Insulin is released into the blood and helps to regulate the amount of glucose (sugar) in the bloodstream. Diabetes is a condition where this process does not function correctly. The reason why diabetes occurs is because no insulin is being produced (often called Type 1 Diabetes) and requires the sufferer to use insulin injections, or insulin is produced but the body becomes resistant to it. This renders the insulin ineffective. This is normally called Type 2 Diabetes and is rapidly becoming more common. The danger is that while diabetes is not immediately life threatening the long term effects of high blood sugar can be damaging to one's health. Uncontrolled diabetes and prolonged high blood sugar levels can, in later life, cause problems to many organs including the kidneys, eyes, nerves and the heart.

This may sound grim, however controlling blood sugar by a combination of medicine, diet and exercise will vastly reduce the long term complications. Recent research shows that 2 in every 100 people have diabetes. Alarmingly half of these people do not even know they have it. Many people have diabetes without being aware of it because someone with diabetes looks no different from anyone else.

How do you find out if you have diabetes? The simplest way to check if you have diabetes is to arrange a blood sugar check with your doctor. A tiny sample of blood, obtained by pricking a finger is checked using a small electronic tester. A normal blood sugar level is generally between 72—126 mg/dl or 4—7 mmol/l (where 1 mmol/l = 18mg/dl). If the body is unable to keep the blood sugar level within these limits, then diabetes is diagnosed. Diagnosis of diabetes can occur out of the blue during a routine check-up but more often it follows from the sufferer experiencing the "symptoms" of diabetes. These symptoms can be many or few, mild or severe depending on the individual. Common Diabetes Symptoms:

Loss Of Weight—Glucose is the form of sugar which is the body's main fuel. Diabetics cannot process this properly so it passes into the urine and out of the body. Less fuel means the body's reserve tissues are broken down to produce energy with a resultant loss in weight.

Thirst—Often it seems no matter how much you drink your mouth still feels dry. The problem is compounded before diabetes is diagnosed by sufferers drinking huge amounts of sugary drinks! Of course this only increases the blood sugar level and leads to increased thirst. Urinating More Often—Sufferers need to urinate often and pass large volumes each time. In addition this symptom takes no account of time so sleep is constantly disturbed by having to visit the bathroom during the night. It is a mistake to think this is caused by the increased thirst and drinking more. On the other hand, high sugar levels in the blood spill over into the urine making it syrupy. To counter-act this water is drawn from the body causing dehydration and therefore thirst. If you have experienced any of these symptoms it does not necessarily follow that you are diabetic however it might be advisable to visit your doctor to be sure. If it does turn out that you have diabetes please do not panic! It can come as a shock and it will mean some changes in your life. While it is incurable it can be treated so the long term complications are reduced or even eliminated. By knowing exactly what diabetes is—and recognizing the symptoms early on—you can prevent it from ever building up within you. Start today by monitoring your health and daily eating habits. Or as they say, preventing is better than finding a cure later on!

Certain factors that contribute to the development of diabetes are. Heredity. Heredity is a major factor. That diabetes can be inherited has been known for centuries. However, the pattern of inheritance is not fully understood. Statistic indicates that those with a family history of the disease have a higher risk of developing diabetes than those without such a background. The risk factor is 25 to 33 percent more. One reason why diabetes, especially type-2 diabetes runs in the family is because of the diabetes gene. But even it is caused by genetic factors beyond your control; there is no reason to suffer from it. Diabetes mellitus cannot be cured in full sense of the term, but it can be effectively controlled so that you would not know the difference. Diet Diabetes has been described by most medical scientists as a prosperity' disease, primarily caused by systematic overeating. Not only is eating too much sugar and refined carbohydrates harmful, but proteins and fats, which are transformed into sugar, may also result in diabetes if taken in excess. It is interesting to note that diabetes is almost unknown in countries where people are poor and cannot afford to overeat. The incidence of diabetes is directly linked with the consumption of processed foods rich in refined carbohydrates, like biscuits, bread, cakes chocolates, pudding and ice creams.

Obesity

Obesity is one of the main causes of diabetes. Studies show that 60 to 85 % of diabetics tend to be overweight. In the United States of America, about 80 percent of type—2 non-insulin dependent dia-betics are reported to be overweight. Excess fat prevents insulin from working properly. The more fatty tissue in the body, the more resistant the muscle and tissue cells become to body insulin. Insulin allows the sugar in the blood to enter the cells by acting on the receptor sites on the surface of the cells. Older people often tend to gain weight, and the same time, many of them develop and mild form of diabetes because who are over weight can often improve their blood sugar simply by losing weight.

Stress and Tension

There is a known connection between stress and diabetes mellitus, those who are under stress and/or lead an irregular lifestyle, need to take adequate precautions and make necessary lifestyle adjustments. Grief, worry and anxiety resulting from examinations, death of a close relative, loss of a joy, business failure and strained marital relationship, all a deep influence on the metabolism and may cause sugar to appear in the urine.

Smoking

Smoking is another important risk factor. Among men who smoke, the risk of developing diabetes is doubled. In women who smoke 25 or more cigarettes a day, the risk of developing diabetes is increased by 40 percent.

Lifestyle Risk

People who are less active have greater risk of developing diabetes. Modern conveniences have made work easier. Physical activity and exercise helps control weight, uses up a lot of glucose (sugar) present in the blood as energy and makes cells more sensitive to insulin. Consequently, the workload on the pancreas is reduced. Diabetes is the fifth-deadliest disease. Since 1987 the death rate has increased 45 percent. in 2002; diabetes claimed an astonishing 224,092 lives in the United States alone. It is believed that the number was actually higher since most deaths of the elderly had multiple chronic conditions associated with their death including diabetes. Many people do not know that they have diabetes until they develop other life threatening conditions such as, heart disease, high blood pressure, blindness, kidney damage, nervous system damage, dental disease, sexual dysfunction, and a number of other complications. When you have diabetes the above complication are side illnesses, diabetes is this root of all of your medical problems and must be under control for you to recover from the side illnesses period! Being checked by your physician on a regular basis is absolutely necessary for your overall quality of life. If you do not know that you have diabetes, there is no other way of knowing that you have this deadly disease without a check up.. While an estimated 14 million people have been diagnosed with diabetes it is also estimated that close to 6.2 million are unaware that they have this deadly disease. In 2005 1.5 million new cases were diagnosed in people age 20 and above. If this dangerous trend continues it is believed that 1 in 3 Americans will develop diabetes in their lifetime. It is also estimated that 41 million Americans have pre-diabetes today. Pre-diabetes is a dangerous condition in itself, this is when the glucose level in the blood is not high enough to be diagnosed as diabetes yet damage is being done to your internal organs. The body can not handle any unsafe level of sugar or glucose in the blood for any extended period of time.

Diabetes is the body's inability to use the sugar called glucose. Glucose is created when the body breaks down food for energy. The hormone insulin opens up the cells in the body to allow glucose to enter into the cell and be used as fuel. In diabetes the cell never opens up and the glucose flows through the blood stream causing high blood sugar levels. With diabetes the body either dose not make enough insulin or is resistant to its own natural insulin. High blood sugar can lead to very serious complications. Heart disease is the leading cause of premature death in people with diabetes. Diabetes is the major cause of leg and foot amputations in Americans today. Infections are much harder to control in people with diabetes, they are at greater risk of complications and death due to infection. The high risk factors leading to type 2 diabetes is too much body fat and high sugar intake!

Diabetes is on the rise; Americans are eating poorly and are lacking physical activity and this is starting to really show in the children of America.

Free-radicals are very active in a person with diabetes. They attack a number of cells at once because diabetes causes an abnormal immune function due to high glucose levels in the blood and organs. Free-radicals are the reason you see so many different complications or side illnesses in this disease. Free-radicals are molecules or atoms that are missing an electron, free-radicals attack healthy cells trying to steal an electron from them. Chronic inflammation is also a major player with this disease and in the side illnesses. Chronic inflammation is being called the silent killer by doctors and scientists. All of the above diseases need medications to help regulate the disease, but you need to know this, medications cause free-radical damage, and this damage is called side effects. All medications can cause side effects. So eating properly to help your condition is absolutely essential for your life.

Think of free-radicals as a school of piranha, they feed on everything in sight, they are not picky eaters. Free-radicals cause healthy cells to become mutated or deformed and they attack any cell they come in contact with. Now if they do manage to steal an electron then that once healthy cell, in turn, becomes a free-radical doing what was done to it

This is a vicious cycle, basically there is a war going on inside your body. You can not see or feel this war but it is there, and one day it will show its ugly head in the form of a serious disease or illness. You must be on the defensive and feed your body what it needs in order to combat these little piranhas.

Inflammation is a bully, after the free-radicals have done the damage the inflammation is sent by the body to help heal but it is unable to heal mutations and deformities so the deformed or mutated cells begin to feed on the healthy inflammation cells. Now the inflammation cells are deformed or mutated and become chronic inflammation cells, the chronic inflammation cells begin attacking your healthy tissues and cells.

You have the power to take your health into your own hands and put a stop to the damage now. As we know anti-oxidants help the body fight against free-radicals, anti-oxidants are molecules or atoms that has an extra electron. It gives this extra electron away and in turn the free-radicals stop attacking healthy cells. Science has proven that ALL diseases and illnesses are caused by free-radical damage and the vast majority have chronic inflammation as their side kick. There are risk factors for all diseases but free-radicals and chronic inflammation are the source and cause of major complications. Free-radicals can not be avoided; they are in air and water pollution, in the junk foods we eat, and caused by traumas and injuries. Free-radicals are a part of life; they even affect the aging process itself. Anti-oxidants are essential for health, plants contain about 1,000 to 1,500 anti-oxidants, a diet of fruits and vegetables is essential, supplements are key, vitamins and minerals contain high numbers of anti-oxidants. You need to do some research and try to find fresh supplements; they tend to lose their potency the longer they sit on the self.

Anyone with diabetes or even pre-diabetes must rethink their diets, moving towards fresh and properly cooked foods, stay away from fast foods and anything with high sugar content. Taking in a large number of anti-oxidants everyday, is essential to help your body recover and maintain better overall health. Type 2 diabetes can be controlled with diet and exercise, as long as you begin now. Pre-diabetes can be reversed. There are also super charged, super powerful anti-oxidants in nature called Xanthones. Xanthones have the power to defeat a larger number of free-radicals at one time, due to strong carbon bonds that make the molecule stable. Each Xanthone performs a specific biological function inside the body unlike regular anti-oxidants.

Universities and scientists have been studying xanthones for over 20 years. Scientists have found that xanthones are able to relieve a variety of problems and also help in the improvement of serious conditions. This is the reason that more and more universities and scientists are becoming involved in the research on these amazing xanthones. People with diabetes are ruled by their medications and checking their blood everyday, they must see their doctor on a regular basis in order to keep their blood sugars under control by adjusting their medication. If their sugar goes too far up or too far down, massive damage to the internal organs and tissues is done and even the brain is affected, and can cause comma. This is a very deadly disease, but with the right food intake it dose not have to be, take care of your self.

What if you are diagnosed with diabetes? Are you going to stay indoors and just inject yourself with insulin everyday? Maybe you need to understand the facts about diabetes and accept it wholeheartedly so that it can't be a heavy burden in your part . Let us start from defining what diabetes really is and the probable causes that brings this disease. Diabetes is a disorder which is the misuse of the digested food for growth and energy by our body. The food that we take in is broken down into glucose, the simplest form of sugar in our blood.

Glucose is the main source of energy of our body. And diabetes actually causes the glucose to back up in our bloodstream, and as more of it is present in our bloodstream, our blood sugar can rise too high.. So understanding the facts about this disease is important, so that the person affected can sustain his life throughout, despite the presence of diabetes. This allows you to live a full and enjoyable life.

African Americans And Diabetes

According to the National Diabetes Education Program, there is a current epidemic of diabetes among African Americans. African Americans are one of the largest groups in the population in the United States that are contracting Type II diabetes. In addition, diabetes is also one of the leading causes of death and disability among African Americans in the United States.

There are certain factors that are believed to cause Type II diabetes, which accounts for nearly 95 percent of all cases of the disease. The causes are generally someone with a close relative with the disease, being an African American or being overweight. Other factors include having high blood pressure, high cholesterol and having gestational diabetes while pregnant. It is estimated that about 3.2 million African Americans have Type II diabetes and about one third of them are undiagnosed.

No one is quite sure why African Americans are more likely to get Type II diabetes than any other ethnic group. One thing is certain, however. Poor African Americans are more likely to die from complications of the disease than those in other ethnic groups. This is most likely due to poor health care in certain communities, limited access to drugs that can potentially save their lives and less education. Affluent African Americans have the same chance as other ethnic groups of dying from complications of the disease.

Many people who live in poor communities, in addition to receiving substandard medical care, little education about disease and limited access to lifesaving drugs, also are inundated with fast food restaurants that seem to target certain ethnic groups. Fast foods are usually very high in carbohydrates, fats and offer very little in the way of nutrition. They are inexpensive, however, and many people with little money find this to be the only way they can feed their family on a limited budget. Unfortunately, most of the foods found in fast food restaurants, particularly French fries, are at the top of the Glycemic Index when it comes to foods that should not be consumed by diabetics. French fries are pretty much the staple of any fast food restaurant. They are high in carbohydrates, high in fat and low in protein. But they are filling.

African Americans can prevent acquiring Type II diabetes in many different ways. One way is to take a look at the Glycemic Index and realize which foods are harmful to them and which to avoid. Another way is to start an exercise regime and, if they are overweight, lose some of those excess pounds. If they are without health care, they should contact their local municipality about screening tests for diabetes. Many clinics and health care facilities offer screening tests for diabetes for those with low income for free. This small step may end up saving the life of someone who is on the verge of getting this potentially life threatening illness.

African Americans can also start saying no to fast foods that, in addition to being precursors for diabetes, are also linked to heart disease, high cholesterol and even cancer.

Many fast food restaurants prey on people in low income areas without regard for the health of those individuals. African Americans need to realize that they are experiencing an epidemic of Type II diabetes in their community and do all that they can to stamp it out.

Depression And Diabetes

Many people who are diagnosed with diabetes are overwhelmed with an onslaught of new information, medications, doctor visits and a feeling of helplessness. Diabetes can be frightening, particularly for anyone who is not familiar with the disease. We read about complications and insulin and medication and feel hopeless.

Many diabetics experience a period of denial when first diagnosed with diabetes. They refuse to believe there is anything wrong with them. While they remain in denial, the condition worsens. This can often lead to depression. Depression and diabetes often go hand in hand. According to the American Diabetes Association, people with diabetes have a greater risk for developing depression than other individuals.

The stress of management of diabetes can take a toll on an individual. There are new medications to take, blood sugar must be monitored frequently and a record kept for your doctor. There are frequent doctor visits and there may be several different medication combinations needed before your blood sugar is kept under control.

On top of that, people who have diabetes are often faced with sudden lifestyle changes. Foods that they once enjoyed are now taboo. An exercise regime is often recommended, which can be good for depression, but people with depression often have little energy to begin an exercise regime. As the depression continues, people often lose interest in monitoring their blood sugar levels and may even skip their medication.

Symptoms of depression include a loss of pleasure in every day activities you used to enjoy as well as a change in appetite. You may have trouble concentrating and have trouble sleeping. Or you may even sleep too much. Many people suffer from depression, but for a diabetic, it can be life threatening. Depression and diabetes is a dangerous combination.

People who are diagnosed with diabetes can empower themselves by learning as much about the disease as possible from the beginning. This can alleviate the feeling of helplessness that often accompanies the diagnoses. Ask your physician questions. Do research. Find out how you can help manage you disease.

If you feel you are suffering from some of the signs of depression, ask your doctor to recommend a therapist who is familiar in dealing with people with chronic illness. Therapy can be crucial for a diabetic patient who feels isolated because of all of the extra work involved in treating their illness. Do not be afraid to discuss your illness with family and friends. Diabetes is a nothing to be ashamed of, it is a disease that affects millions of people.

If at all possible, join a support group for others who also have diabetes. Here you can not only find kindred spirits who are experiencing some of the same fears as yourself, but you can also learn new information.

Any time someone is diagnosed with an illness puts them at risk for depression. Their world has changed and no longer feels safe. Worse of all, they feel out of control. If you are diagnosed with diabetes, take back the control and learn how to manage your disease. By empowering yourself, you will not only be able to effectively manage your diabetes, you will eliminate the depression.

Diabetes And Sexual Problems

As if people with diabetes do not have enough to worry about, they also have to contend with sexual problems. Diabetes and sexual problems affect both men and women but in different ways. Because your body responds to sexual stimuli through your nerves and high blood glucose levels affect your nervous system, it is understandable that even sexual response is affected by this potentially life threatening condition.

In men, diabetes and sexual problems often focus on erectile dysfunction. It is estimated by the American Diabetes Institute that as many as 85 percent of men with diabetes experience erectile dysfunction. This can cause problems in marriage but, more importantly, can cause severe depression in those who are contending not only with the disease of diabetes, but also what they deem the loss of their self esteem.

Erectile dysfunction can also be a symptom of diabetes. If a man continues to experience this malady, he should discuss this problem with his physician to make sure that he is not suffering from undiagnosed diabetes. Fortunately, there are certain medications and other treatments available to men who experience this common side effect to diabetes. The key to eliminating the problem is for the patient to discuss this with his physician.

Diabetes and sexual problems does not stop at erectile dysfunction, however. Retrograde ejaculation is a more potentially dangerous situation that can happen to men with diabetes. In this condition, the semen can go into the bladder instead of being dispelled out of the penis during ejaculation. A man who is experiencing this side effect of diabetes should seek consultation with a urologist who can help with medication or surgery to correct the problem.

Men are not the only ones affected with sexual problems as a side effect to diabetes. Diabetes and sexual problems also affect women. Because of damage to the nerve cells within the vagina by high levels of blood glucose, dryness can occur that can make intercourse very painful. Many women also report that the nerve damage caused by the hyperglycemia also causes them to lose interest in sex and have no sensations in their genital area. Needless to say, the lack of sexual desire can cause psychological problems for both men and women and may lead to marital difficulties as well.

Many people are embarrassed about speaking to their physician when it comes to problems relating to sexual relations. People with diabetes should be aware of the fact that their condition makes them prone to these side effects and should discuss them with their doctor so they can get treatment. There is a variety of treatment for those experiencing diabetes and sexual problems.

One way to prevent such problems from occurring is to maintain your blood glucose levels by eating a healthy diet, exercising and taking your prescribed medication or insulin. Monitor your blood sugars as instructed by your physician. If you experience any side effects related to your condition, discuss them with your physician. By keeping informed of the disease and the side effects as well as complications, you can empower yourself in managing your illness and lead a happier as well as longer life.

The X Factor: How Fast Can It Ruin Your Life?

It was absolutely embarrassing! I couldn't stay awake. After eating a normal breakfast lunch or dinner I was out like a light. No I am not talking about the Thanksgiving turkey tryptophan thing that is the brunt of so many jokes-this was not funny at all.

I tried to cope with this for over a year until one day driving in town on a busy street in broad daylight- I fell asleep at the wheel. That was bad enough but as it happened my fiancée was with me to witness the event. Fortunately the worst that happened was I scared the hell out of both of us. That did it- I had to get some help.

I went to see a health practitioner who knew immediately what I had-Syndrome X.

I still remember going home to see what else I could find out about Syndrome X besides the take home literature which was very scant. It was not a common term for sure. There just wasn't much information out there in 1995.

In a nutshell this ominous sounding term refers to a group of symptoms centered on insulin resistance. Without making it too confusing I'll try to explain.

After a meal someone with Syndrome X will have elevated glucose in the blood which signals the pancreas to make more insulin. This forces the blood sugar down, which can lead to food cravings, which can lead to—you guessed it- OBESITY and a host of other serious problems like hypertension, high triglycerides, diabetes, and coronary heart disease.

Syndrome X interferes with the body's ability to burn food. Muscle cells become more resistant to insulin thus reducing the ability to absorb nutrients which in turn causes the pancreas to produce more insulin. Got it? Let me try again.

If you have Syndrome X your body's metabolism is screwed up (not a medical term). It causes you to have food cravings notably for sweets (sugar) and bread and pasta (white flour) to a point of almost being addictive. Can you see where this is headed?

Some think that Syndrome X is actually caused by eating too many high carb foods like bread, pasta and sweets. As many as 75 million Americans have Syndrome X in one degree or another. Sure is a good thing I wasn't a snackaholic, chocaholic, or addicted to pasta and bread.

Is it any coincidence at all that the prevalence of Syndrome X, pre-diabetes, and obesity in all age groups-especially children-has something to do with the much more serious problems of diabetes, hypertension, higher triglycerides, and CHD?

That's the bad news! The good news is that the more serious problems can all be prevented. Weight loss of up to 15 % of your current weight will have an impact on lowering your blood pressure and raising your HDL or good cholesterol. A diet low in refined carbs such as soda, high fructose corn syrup, sugar and white flour bread and pasta will help with weight loss and getting your triglycerides down. And of course exercise-even a 30 minute walk a day can do wonders.

So be good to yourself, your spouse and children; lose the weight, exercise, and change your diet. If you don't the evil downward spiral of Syndrome X will ruin your life.

Quick Guide To Understanding Your Cholesterol

Cholesterol is a fatlike substance which is found in the tissue of humans and other animals. It plays important roles in cell membrane structure, certain hormones, and manufacturing vitamin D. Our livers procude all of the cholesterol that we need for these important functions. Excess cholesterol can contribute to antherosclerosis or clogging of the arteries.

Cholesterol is found in all food from animal sources: meat, eggs, fish, poultry, and dairy products. Some animal foods contribute substantial amounts of cholesterol, while others contribute only small amounts. There is no cholesterol in any plant-derived foods. Excess dietary cholesterol can increase blood cholesterol, which can increase the risk of coronary heart disease.

You'll often hear cholesterol referred to as either good cholesterol or bad cholesterol. To help in our understanding of the two and their differences, we first need to define the word "lipoproteins." These are packets of proteins, cholesterol, and triglycerides that are assembled by the liver and circulated in the blood. When we talk about LDL cholesterol, we're referring to low density lipoprotein cholesterol. And when we refer to HDL cholesterol, we're referring to high density lipoprotein cholesterol.

LDL cholesterol, often referred to as "bad cholesterol," carried cholesterol through the bloodstream, dropping it off where it's needed for cell building and leaving behind any unused residue of cholesterol as plague on the walls of the arteries.

HDL cholesterol, often referred to as "good cholesterol," picks up the cholesterol which has been deposited in the arteries and brings it back to the liver for reprocessing or excretion.

You can easily understand why there's a distinction between good and bad cholesterol now that you understand the unique functions of each.

Saturated fats are usually from animal products such as lard, fats in meat and chicken skin, butter, ice cream, milk fat, cheese, etc. Tropical oils such as coconut oil and palm oil are also highly saturated. These fats are usually solid at room temperature. You've undoubtedly heard from somewhere that you should keep your saturated fats to a minimum, but do you know why? Because these fats tend to increase your blood cholesterol levels, which in turn increases your risk of coronary heart disease.

Hydrogenated fats are those liquid vegetable oils than have been turned into solid saturated fats through a chemical process. These fats also contribute to your blood cholesterol levels.

Polyunsaturated fats are liquid at room temperature and derived from plants. Examples: safflower, corn, soybean, cottenseed and sunflower oils. Polyunsaturated fats tend to lower LDL (your bad cholesterol), but in excess can also lower your HDL (good cholesterol).

Monounsaturated fats are also derived from plants. These include olive oils and canola oil. Replacing the saturated fats in your diet with monounsaturated fats can help to lower your LDL (again, bad cholesterol) without lowering your HDL (good cholesterol). This is why monounsaturated fats are a healthy choice for your heart. However, keep in mind that too much of any form of fat can contribute to obesity.

The bottomline: whenever you're making a choice about the fats you use, keep in mind that good heart health depends on keeping your LDL cholesterol low while maintaining your HDL cholesterol.

More Aware Of Diabetes-Heart Disease Link

With diabetes on the rise, doctors are extremely concerned about associated risks such as heart disease and stroke, which together kill two out of three people with diabetes. Fortunately, a recent study indicates that more people with diabetes are making the link between diabetes and their increased risk for heart disease and stroke.

According to a 2005 awareness survey conducted by the American Diabetes Association (ADA) and American College of Cardiology (ACC), 45 percent of people with diabetes understand their increased risk for heart disease, which is up from 35 percent in 2001.

Experts believe even more awareness is needed, however. The ADA and ACC continue to work together to share important information, tools and resources to encourage people with diabetes-and health care providers-to learn more about the impact of diabetes on the heart.

Other findings from the 2005 ADA/ACC awareness survey show:

• 69 percent know they may develop high blood pressure (38 percent in 2001).

• 64 percent know they are at risk for cholesterol problems (37 percent in 2001).

Importantly, more people with diabetes are talking to their health care providers about managing diabetes comprehensively:

• 45 percent of people with diabetes now have a goal for blood glucose levels (30 percent in 2003).

• 57 percent have a goal for blood pressure (34 percent in 2003).

• 61 percent have a goal for cholesterol (34 percent in 2003).
Title:

What Exactly Is This "Gestational Diabetes"?

Gestational diabetes is a temporary condition that occurs during pregnancy. It is one of the top health complications that a woman has to face during pregnancy. Indeed a double curse!

If the woman had gestational diabetes during pregnancy then she is most likely to pass it on to the child. So, if a woman has gestational diabetes during pregnancy, there is an increased risk of developing diabetes for both mother and child. Timely knowledge about this condition, goes to control it effectively by diet and exercise. After the baby is born, the mother and the child both recoup their original health.

One problem gives room for a series of problems. The major risk is the birth of a fat baby. The condition is known as macrosomia. The baby by birth will have its own problems, the common one being damage to its shoulders during birth.

Some basic precautions have to be taken to prevent the risk of gestational diabetes. It is taking recourse to natural methods again! Make it a point to lose weight, if you are overweight. Be careful and choosy about your food, and above all, do exercises regularly. This type of diabetes is a temporary condition, a passing phase, that occurs during pregnancy.

There is another risk for the baby. It may develop breathing problems.

The exact causes of the gestational diabetes are not known yet. But there are certain clues and possibilities, why gestational diabetes occurs! It is insulin resistance.

The baby, as it grows, is supported by the placenta. Hormones help the baby develop. But the hormones also do a damaging act. They block the action of the mother's insulin in her body. The mother's body finds it hard to use insulin, so her requirement of insulin goes up by 300 % and gestational diabetes is the result!

Utmost care is needed to combat gestational diabetes, as it concerns the health of the mother as well as that of the baby. Food choices are of paramount importance. This will have beneficial effects on the health of your baby's growth. If you are fit and healthy, the risk of cesarean section birth can also be avoided.

In many cases, it has been found that gestational diabetes leads to type II diabetes later.

Do exercises regularly even during pregnancy, but only after consulting your doctor. This is the formative period for you as well as for the baby. Proper exercises provide strength to your body and act favorably for the growth of the baby within.

Shut the door on the face of the diabetes, even if it pleads that it is only gestation. This evil does not deserve mercy.

These figures are encouraging, but awareness may not be moving fast enough to keep pace with the growing prevalence of diabetes.

Recent statistics indicate diabetes has risen by over 14 percent since last estimates in 2003. The need for increased education and awareness about the link between diabetes and heart disease is now more critical than ever.

Armed with the best information, people with diabetes can properly manage their diabetes, understand their risks for complications such as heart disease and stroke, and take action to live a longer, healthier life.

Chapter II
Symptoms

Having diabetes can change the life of person entirely. From the way one chooses the foods that he will eat to the way he lives his daily life, everything will change. For someone who doesn't know much about diabetes there are a lot of webs sites, magazines, and books that can help you understand better of the nature of diabetes.

The greatest problem for diabetics is not being able to access medication when emergency situations occur. That is why, it is important to always have an emergency kit at hand. To keep the medicines from expiring, use them from time to time and replace them with new refills. The emergency kit can include cold medications, antacids, cough syrup, test strips and insulin with syringes if you use one and blood glucose monitoring supplies. If you will purchase over the counter medicines, make sure to read the label before using it. If there is a warning that diabetic people should consult their doctor before using the product, then do so. If you have these emergency kits at home, try to also have it at work or at school.It is also essential to include in the emergency kit your medical history, prescription medications and emergency contacts. To keep them from getting wet, keep them in a water proof bags. If you are using insulin keep extra syringes, glucagons emergency kit and urine ketone strips. A glucagon emergency kit consists of a syringe filled with liquid which must be mixed with a powder. This kit is only used in case of a Severe Hypoglycemic Emergency. Try also to keep the insulin in a cool place as much as possible to keep it from being damaged. For people who got caught in the Katrina and Rita hurricane disaster, being prepared made the difference between life and death. And for people with diabetes, being prepared is important to their own personal safety and health. Hence, the best thing a diabetic person can do to prevent any problem with diabetes is to live a healthy lifestyle. It is important to eat healthy foods and have a regular exercise to keep blood pressures at normal and reduce the risk of heart disease and other serious conditions. And most importantly, have emergency kits close at hand at all times.

Diagnosing diabetes symptoms can be difficult in identifying at first, as manifestation of the disease is gradual. Sometimes, because symptoms can also be common to other illnesses, the real illness may be overlooked. Diabetes symptoms may vary, the list may go on and on but not everybody (diabetes patients) has them.

There are even some cases that no symptoms may show on some patients. Diabetes occurs when the body's ability to react to insulin gets affected. The insulin is your body hormone that allows your blood sugar (glucose) to enter body cells. When too much glucose enters the blood, this leads to the elevated amount of blood glucose, which it can cause glucose spillage towards the urine. This is the primary reason why one of the most classic diabetes symptoms, frequent urination, plagues the patient.

Because elevated glucose level is beyond normal, your body cells are energy-starved and consequently leading to the damage in your nerves, kidneys, eyes, blood vessels and your heart. The increased amount of glucose appears when the sugar of your body falls too low. It then increases production of sugar. This process starts when the pancreas releases the hormone called glucagons. The stored glycogen will be converted back into the glucose by your liver and muscles.

How are diabetes symptoms diagnosed? Diagnosing diabetes patients may vary, and is based according to the duration and range of the high blood sugar levels. Patients with type 2 diabetes are often diagnosed relatively slowly as compared to people with type 1 diabetes, to which it may take only after weeks or some months. Symptoms may also progress slowly and mildly.

Some of the most specific and common early diabetes symptoms are:

- Skin irritation and diseases
- Skin infections
- Poor skin healing
- Athlete's foot
- Sexual problem
- Unusual vaginal dryness
- Erectile failure (to male patients)
- Premature menopause (to female patients)
- Absence of menstrual periods
- Paresthesias

- Peripheral neuropathy
- Urinary tract infection
- Blurry vision
- Malaise
- Drowsiness
- Numbness of the hands
- Weight loss or weight gain

Other more extreme diabetes symptoms are:

- Excessive urination
- Excessive thirstiness
- Dehydration
- Weight loss even with an increased appetite
- Tiredness, fatigue, nausea, and vomiting
- Excessive hunger
- More bladder, skin and vaginal infections
- Serious blurry vision
- Headache
- Muscle aches, weakness and cramps
- Acne
- Increased sexual problems because of erectile failure for men, and vaginal dryness for women
- Cessation of menstrual periods

Other diabetes symptoms:

- Gums are bleeding
- Unusual noise or buzzing in the ear
- Feet numbness or tingling
- Skin itching

- Diarrhea
- Confusion

Depression

Complications associated to diabetes symptoms:

- Kidney diseases
- Diabetic retinopathy
- Sciatica

Heart diseases and
- Stroke

As those mentioned symptoms might occur at a later time for a patient, the usual situation is delayed scheduling of the check-up. This is not a good idea as complications may increase over time, making it even harder to treat and manage the disease. In this case, it is extremely important to check with the doctor in as early as possible to prevent more damage to the body. Another, it is important to note that diabetes is one of the lifelong diseases, and one that does not infect other people upon contact.

Diagnosing diabetes symptoms can be difficult in identifying at first, as manifestation of the disease is gradual. Sometimes, because symptoms can also be common to other illnesses, the real illness may be overlooked. Diabetes symptoms may vary, the list may go on and on but not everybody (diabetes patients) has them. There are even some cases that no symptoms may show on some patients.

Diabetes occurs when the body's ability to react to insulin gets affected. The insulin is your body hormone that allows your blood sugar (glucose) to enter body cells. When too much glucose enters the blood, this leads to the elevated amount of blood glucose, which it can cause glucose spillage towards the urine.

As those mentioned symptoms might occur at a later time for a patient, the usual situation is delayed scheduling of the check-up. This is not a good idea as complications may increase over time, making it even harder to treat and manage the disease. In this case, it is extremely important to check with the doctor in as early as possible to prevent more damage to the body. Another, it is important to note that diabetes is one of the lifelong diseases, and one that does not infect other people upon contact.

Could You Have Diabetes-And Not Know it?

Take this test to see if you are at risk for having diabetes. Diabetes is more common in African Americans, Latinos, Native Americans, Asian Americans and Pacific Islanders. If you are a member of one of these ethnic groups, you need to pay special attention to this test. Write in the points next to each statement that is true for you. If a statement is not true, put a zero. Then add your total score.

1. I am a woman who has had a baby weighing more than nine pounds at birth. Yes I _____

2. I have a sister or brother with diabetes. Yes I _____

3. I have a parent with diabetes. Yes I _____

4. My weight is equal to or above that listed in the chart.
Yes 5 _____

I am under 65 years of age and I get little or no exercise.
Yes 5_____

6. I am between 45 and 64 years of age.
Yes 5 _____ 7. I am 65 years old or older.

Yes 9 _____TOTAL Scoring 10 or more points: You are at high risk for having diabetes. Only your health care provider can check to see if you have diabetes. See yours soon and find out for sure. Scoring 3 to 9 points: You are probably at low risk for having diabetes now. But don't just forget about it. Keep your risk low by losing weight if you are overweight, being active most days and eating low-fat meals that are high in fruits and vegetables and whole grain foods. Diabetes is a serious disease that can lead to blindness, heart disease, strokes, kidney failure and loss of a limb.

The onset of Type 2 diabetes is often very gradual and may develop without any symptoms at all. Sadly, the diagnosis most often is made only after a complication of the disease happens. Acupuncture. Acupuncture is a procedure in that a practitioner inserts needles into designated points on the skin. Some Western scientists believe that acupuncture triggers the release of the body's natural painkillers. Acupuncture has been shown to offer relief from chronic pain. Acupuncture is sometimes used by people with neuropathy, the painful nerve damage of diabetes. Your weight affects your health in many ways. Being overweight can keep your body from making and using insulin. I think I had it for about three years before I realized it. How serious is Diabetes? Very! The early symptoms of untreated diabetes mellitus are related to the elevated blood glucose levels.

Pre Diabetes

Type II Diabetes has become somewhat of an epidemic of late. More and more people are being diagnosed with this potentially life threatening condition. Type II Diabetes usually sets on later in life, although more younger people are being diagnosed every day with this disease.

According to the American Diabetes Association, approximately 54 million people in the United States have pre diabetes. Pre diabetes is a condition in which the blood glucose levels are higher than normal but not high enough to be considered Type II diabetes. Although pre diabetes is not a full fledged disease, it can also cause complications in the heart and blood circulation if left untreated.

The good news about pre diabetes is that with proper nutrition and the care of a physician, you can avoid being diagnosed with Type II diabetes. The condition can reverse itself, but it does take work on the part of the individual, as well as compliance with the orders directed by your physician.

Obesity is also an epidemic in the United States and many in the medical community believe that this is contributory to the corresponding diabetic epidemic. It is the general consensus of the medical community that obesity is a precursor to Type II diabetes. Therefore, those who have pre diabetes can stave off the disease by making some healthy life choices that will eliminate their need for medication or insulin in later years.

One way to reverse the effects of pre diabetes is to maintain a healthy weight. This can be easily accomplished through diet and exercise. For those who feel that it is too much trouble to manage their weight or complain that they do not have the time to exercise, they need to realize that the time they spend exercising now can eliminate their time spent on dialysis. While not all people with diabetes experience kidney failure, many do. And when the kidneys fail, these patients must spend many hours each week, hooked up to a machine that functions as their kidneys.

Those who complain that they do not want to watch their diet can be reminded that it is easier to watch their diet than to inject themselves with insulin or monitor their blood glucose levels several times a day. Those who feel that foods that are rich in carbohydrates are less expensive than healthier alternatives can be reminded of the cost of medications and doctor visits for those who refuse to take control of their condition right away.

While some people are pre disposed to diabetes through genetic factors, others acquire this disease by eating too many bad carbohydrates, being inactive and not maintaining a healthy weight. If you have been told that you have pre diabetes, do not fret. You can reverse this condition. Begin an exercise regime, even if it only entails walking. Take a look at the Glycemic Index that explains which foods diabetics should avoid and follow these suggestions.

See your doctor about being put on a weight loss program and make certain that he or she continues to monitor your blood glucose levels. Pre diabetes does not have to turn into Type II diabetes. By developing a healthier lifestyle, you can reverse this condition and lead a longer, healthier life.

Teeth Complications of Diabetes

People who suffer from diabetes must be extra vigilant when it comes to taking care of their teeth. Diabetics do not process sugars and starches from their systems effectively and this causes their blood glucose levels to remain high. The condition of high blood glucose is called glycemia. It can cause many complications in an individual including those that affect the kidneys, heart, blood, eyes, and even the central nervous system. People do not die from diabetes. They die from complications caused by the disease that is often allowed to get out of control.

Everyone is prone to tooth and gum problems. There are many causes. Heredity plays an important role as does dental hygiene. Smoking also contributes to tooth and gum problems. But the diabetic has more of a chance of developing tooth and gum disease than the average person. If a diabetic allows his or her blood glucose level to remain high, it has a severe impact on their teeth. This is particularly true if the person with diabetes is older than 45, an age when many people begin experiencing problems with their teeth.

High blood glucose levels make one more prone to infection. Periodontitis is an infection that affects both the gums and bones in the mouth. People with this condition often have receding gums that make their teeth look larger than they are. A person with diabetes must make certain that he or she receives a dental exam periodically to make certain that they do not acquire this infection of the gums and bones. If left untreated, Periodontitis can cause someone to lose their teeth.

It usually begins with a buildup of germs in the teeth that are helped along with the high blood glucose. One of the problems with having glycemia is that it enables germs to grow faster than they would on someone without this condition. As the germs begin to build up on the teeth and gums, the gums begin to get red and sore and swell. In many times, a person can see that they have gum disease when they brush their teeth and the gums begin to bleed. This is the time you want to call your dentist.

If untreated, the gum disease can lead to the infection of Periodontitis that can become so severe that it causes one to lose their teeth. Many people with diabetes as well as those with compromised immune disorders risk acquiring this disease. This is why it is so important to have your teeth examined by a dentist on a regular basis.

Teeth complications of diabetes do not have to cause one to lose their teeth. If caught early, there are many procedures a dentist can perform to stave off infection and save the teeth. In addition, a person with diabetes can help eliminate teeth complications of diabetes by following the advice of their physician when it comes to controlling their disease. Use the Glycemic Index to understand which foods to avoid that will raise your glucose levels. Exercise and maintain a healthy weight. Do not smoke. Avoid alcohol and take any medication or insulin as prescribed. In addition, it is imperative for a person with diabetes to monitor his or her blood glucose levels periodically throughout the day and keep an accurate record of their readings. This information should be presented to the physician at each visit so he or she knows if your medications need to be changed.

By managing the care of your diabetes, you can avoid many of the complications that accompany this disease. By seeing your dentist on a regular basis and informing him or her of your condition, they can help you with a regiment that will enable you to maintain healthy gums, avoid infection and allow you to keep your teeth.

Chapter III
Choices

It may sound like a hard thing to do—be consistent and have variety in your diet at the same time. But it is possible and it is the best way to control your diabetes with your diet. The consistency comes in at specific meal times and the same servings from the different food groups. And the variety refers to trying as many different foods in the food groups as you can.

It can be easy to find a few meals that work well with your blood sugars and are easy to prepare and just stick with them. You are more than likely to get bored with this and you probably aren't getting all of the nutrients you need from a set amount of foods.

Whether you are on the carbohydrate counting diet or the exchange diet, you have a lot of room for flexibility. You can combine different foods together for something new or try foods you have never had before. You can meet with your dietician to get additional ideas for recipes and other foods that you can eat to add more variety to your diet.

There will be times that you try a new food and your blood sugars are higher as a result. Think back about anything else that you had done differently that day—less activity or taking your insulin later than usual. If the new food is the only change you experienced talk to your dietician. You may be able to prepare the food differently or eat it with something else or you may have to avoid that food if it doesn't work for your diabetic diet.

The glycemic index diet is one that many diabetics find useful. The diet is based on assigning foods a ranking that indicates that food's effect on blood sugar levels. This can be a valuable tool for diabetics, especially ones that have been newly diagnosed as it can take some of the guess work out of meal planning and what foods to eat.

The glycemic index (GI) diet indicates foods that have a low GI value meaning they will take a longer time to have an affect on blood sugars and ones that have a higher value—they will act quicker to raise blood sugars. A diabetic is still going to have to use another means to decide what foods to eat though—such as the food pyramid or an exchange list as not all items on the GI diet are as healthy as they could be. Meaning a food that has a low index does not mean it is a better choice for you than some foods that are on the higher end of the scale.

Using the GI diet as your sole source of meal planning is not recommended not only because the values are not indicative of the healthiest choice but also because not all foods are listed. If you are basing your diet on this method and want to add other foods that do not have GI rating you are not going to be able to properly plan. Until more information is researched on the diet or it is made more comprehensive it should be used with an approved diet for diabetics such as the exchange diet or the carbohydrate counting diet.

If you want more information on how to incorporate the GI diet with your current meal plan, consult with your dietician or a diabetes educator. Just because you have diabetes doesn't mean that you can' be adventurous and try something new, just do it at regular meal times and within the recommended portion sizes.

Reading Food Labels

On all packaged food that you buy, there is a food label that includes important information to a diabetic. You need to learn how to read them properly and know what the different numbers and percentages mean to you and your diabetic diet. Below is an overview of the basic information you need to know about food labels.

Whether you are counting carbohydrates, are following the exchange diet, or you are on the Therapeutic Lifestyle Changes (TLC) diet you can increase your chances for success by reading your food labels and understanding what they mean.

The ingredient list is a good place to start before looking at the numbers in the food label. Where is sugar on the ingredient list? The closer it is to the beginning of the list the more of it is present in the food. That goes the same for all ingredients; manufacturers list the ingredients in order of the amount that is in the product. If there are things in your food that do not work well for your blood sugar on the list it should be avoided or eaten in moderation.

Look at the serving size and compare that to the number of carbohydrates is in a serving. Most servings of carbohydrates for a diabetic are 15 grams. If one serving is higher than 15 grams you will have to eat less than the suggested serving size to stay on track with your meal plan.

Sugar-free foods may grab your attention as something safe and yummy to add to your shopping cart. But look at the carbohydrate count first. Most foods that are made sugar-free using artificial sweeteners and sugar substitutes have higher carbohydrate counts.

Check the fat content too, look for a low percent of your daily intake and ideally it will be monounsaturated as opposed to polyunsaturated or saturated fats.

Benefits of the Exchange Diet

The exchange diet is one that allows you to pick and choose the foods you eat from each of the six food groups based on portion sizes. When you begin eating with this diet, it may seem like a lot of work but as you get used to the portions sizes and the common substitutions that you make it will get easier.

One of the benefits of the exchange diet it the flexibility you have in your meal planning. As long as you are eating the correct number of exchanges from each food group you will maintain better control of your blood glucose levels.

If you get bored quite easily by eating the same food day in and day out, the exchange diet might be for you. There are endless possibilities to combine different foods together at meal times. You can have broccoli for dinner three nights in a row but make it a completely different meal each time. One night you can have one small potato, ½ cup of steamed broccoli and a one ounce pork chop; the second night have ½ cup of cooked pasta tossed with ½ cup of broccoli and one ounce of cooked chicken; and the third night try 1/3 cup of rice mixed with ½ cup of broccoli and one ounce of lean ground beef.

The exchange diet also takes the guess work out of meal planning for diabetics. It is laid out in a very straight forward and easy to understand manner. If there are foods that you cannot find on the exchange list given to you by your dietician, call and find out which group it belongs too and what a proper portion size is.

At first you should weigh and measure your foods to ensure you are using the proper amounts but as time passes you will be able to do this by sight.

When to Eat when you have Diabetes

When you are a diabetic sometimes when you eat is just as important as what you eat. Keeping a steady stream of food in your system without causing high blood sugars can be hard to do. But once you figure what works for you, you will have more flexibility and better control of your diabetes.

It is recommended that diabetics eat many small meals throughout the day or three main meals and three snacks in between. A typical day may go like this:

*   Wake-up and have breakfast
*   Mid-morning snack
*   Lunch
*   Mid-afternoon snack
*   Dinner
*   Bedtime snack

The timing in between each meal or snack should be two to three hours. This variation will depend on what you have eaten at the previous meal, how active you have been and what you feel like. If you are feeling hungry or light-headed and you normally wouldn't have eaten for another 30 minutes—don't wait. Test your blood sugar and move up your meal. The time it can take for you to wait the 30 minutes can be the time it takes for your blood sugar to drop dangerously low.

The only time you may want to wait a longer period of time is between dinner and your bedtime snack. Most times dinner is the biggest meal of the day and you will not need food again for a longer period of time. Another reason to wait longer is to ensure that you have enough food in your system before you go to bed to last you through the night without your blood sugars dropping too low.

If eating this many times in a day is too much for you, consider eating smaller means and smaller portion sizes. Eating this way (less more often) makes it easier for your body to regulate blood glucose levels.

Good Carbohydrates and Bad Carbohydrates

A lot of diabetic diets and diabetic meal planning center around carbohydrate intake—the amount you can have and when you should have them. This is because they play such a crucial role in managing blood sugars. Too many carbohydrates or the wrong kind can cause high blood sugars. Not enough carbohydrates can cause low blood sugars or hypoglycemia.

It is recommended that carbohydrates make up about 40% of your daily calories, but not all carbohydrates are created equal. You also need to pay attention to fat and sugar content.

Here are some carbohydrate choices that should be made frequently:

* Whole grain cereals
* Whole wheat breads and rolls
* Brown rice
* Whole wheat crackers
* Raw or lightly steamed fruits and vegetables
* Whole wheat pita pockets or wraps

Carbohydrate choices that should be made less often:

* Potato chips
* White bread
* White rice
* Other foods that have been processed
* Cookies
* Easy to eat snacks

Carbohydrates are an essential part of every diet but make sure you are including the right kinds in yours. Good carbohydrates will fill you up and not create a sudden spike in your blood sugars. Bad carbohydrates are usually over-processed, create high blood sugars, create obesity and are high in sodium.

As carbohydrates are going to make up almost half of your daily food choices it is important to fill you body with high-quality choices. Choose ones that will give you energy and not cause you to gain weight. The less processed or refined a carbohydrate is the better it is going to be for you. Even when baking, choose unbleached whole grain flour. It doesn't make a big difference in taste but it does in the quality of carbohydrate it creates. Try whole grain flour in pancakes, cookies and cakes.

Low carb diets are very effective in achieving weight loss when followed. But the key word there is that they should be followed. However, there are controversies about their "healthiness". Definitely, people get into these diets to lose weight. But what every person getting into this is not only the aspect of losing weight but also as always, keeping the weight off. But it goes beyond that. It also involves being and staying healthy and functional in whatever we do everyday. A slim person is definitely not attractive if he or she is weak from lack of nutrients and energy due to these low carb diets.

The body uses up carbohydrates first as a source of energy. If there are more carbohydrates taken in, the body stores the surplus as fat. If there are fewer carbohydrates taken it, the body is forced to use the stored fat for its energy requirement.

The Role of Fiber in a Diabetic Diet

The role of fiber in healthy diets is very important—it aids in digestion and keep your colon and other organs healthy and functioning properly. It is also a wonder element that should be a large part of any diabetic's diet. You will reap many benefits from including fiber in your diet. If you are pre-diabetic it can assist in delaying the diagnosis of diabetes or if you are already diabetic it can help keep your blood glucose under control.

Fiber will keep you feeling fuller longer—it slows the conversion of carbohydrates in your body which in turn can keep your blood sugars stable. The type of fiber that a diabetic needs to eat to gain these benefits is soluble fiber (dissolves in water). Some good sources of soluble fiber include:

* Choosing whole grain or whole wheat products instead of white (flour, breads, and cereals)
* Eating fresh fruit and vegetables instead of processed or drinking them in liquid form
* Beans, use dried beans in your favorite recipes like chili for a wholesome, high-fiber meal

To ensure that you are getting the most benefit from eating increased amount of fiber, make sure that you are drinking at least eight glasses of water a day. Remember, this fiber dissolves in water and you need to stay hydrated for it to work properly.

If you are on a carbohydrate counting diet and are using 15 grams of carbohydrates for one serving you can increase the amount you are eating if that item has high-fiber content. You can subtract the number of grams of fiber in a serving from the number of carbohydrates. For instance if you are eating an item that has 20 grams of carbohydrates (over the one serving limit) but it has five grams of fiber you can subtract the five from the twenty and it is now only a 15 gram serving.

The latest dieting craze has no doubt been the low carb high protein diets. Those of you on Atkins, South Beach etc will no doubt have noticed a number of changes since you took up the diet. And no I'm not talking about the remarkable weight loss I am talking about your bad breath. Now it may not have been noticeable to you but I suggest you ask your friends or relatives whether there has been a detioration and you may be surprised by the answer. In fact you may even find your friends moving away from you when you speak which is always a sure sign of bad breath.

So what's the cause of all this bad air? Well depending on which medical speak you speak with there are a number, yet similar, reasons for the problem. One of the reasons is directly related to the increase in protein which most of the low carb diets advocate.

Basically, we all have a large number of useful bacteria living mainly on our tongue and at the back of our throat. These bacteria are supposed to be there, because they assist humans in digestion by breaking down proteins found in specific foods, mucous or phlegm, blood, and in diseased or "broken-down" oral tissue. When these beneficial bacteria come into contact with these compounds, the odorous and "lousy-tasting" volatile sulfur compounds (VSCs') are released from the back of the tongue and throat, as Hydrogen Sulphide, Methyl Mercaptan, and other odorous and bad tasting compounds.

Since the bacteria are meant to be in our mouth there is no way we can remove them permanently. So, no amount of brushing or tongue scraping will get rid of the VSCs'. The only scientifically proven way of curing your bad breath (Halitosis) is by attacking the bacteria's ability to produce VSCs' and by converting the VSC into non-odorous and non-tasting organic salts.

There are a number of ways in which the problem is worsened and the most common way is with dry mouth.

This generally occurs while you are asleep and hence the reason you sometimes wake up with "morning breath".

Although some cases of dry mouth are naturally occurring, most cases are caused by one of these factors:

1. Prescription Medications (usually prescribed for high blood pressure or depression)
2. Antihistamines
3. Adult Beverages
4. Mouthwashes with alcohol in them

When your mouth is dryer, you have less Saliva. Saliva naturally contains Oxygen, which keeps your mouth healthy and fresh. These bacteria are anaerobic, which simply means that they will thrive and make more sulfur in the presence of little or no oxygen. Thus if you have less Saliva, you have less oxygen, thereby creating an anaerobic environment, perfect for the bacteria to produce more of these odorous and sour/bitter compounds. Because of the increase in higher protein foods, on an Atkins type diet, especially dairy products, the amount of Volatile. Sulfur Compounds increases dramatically and as such your breath gets worse accordingly. The only way to fight the problem is to try and supply oxygen to the bacteria causing the problem and remove as much of the VSCs' as possible. This can be done in a number of ways:

Drink loads of water. This will help ensure your tongue and throat are kept moist and supplying oxygen to the VSC producing bacteria.

Always clean your tongue with a tongue cleaner before brushing your teeth last thing at night and first thing in morning. You should also try and do this after every meal too.

- Use a mouthwash which does not contain any alcohol as alcohol can dry your mouth and make the problem worse. You can also dramatically improve matters by using an oxygenating mouthwash. You can find one by doing a Google on "oxygenating mouthwash".
- Don't chew gum, which contains sugar, to try and mask the bad breath. This can make matters worse. Use a sugar free gum instead.

The bottom line is that low carb diets will cause bad breath, although for some it will be a lot worse than others. However, help is at hand so if you want to shed the weight and not shed any friends then make sure and heed the advice given above.

The Glycemic Index and Diabetic Diets

The glycemic index diet is one that many diabetics find useful. The diet is based on assigning foods a ranking that indicates that food's effect on blood sugar levels. This can be a valuable tool for diabetics, especially ones that have been newly diagnosed as it can take some of the guess work out of meal planning and what foods to eat. The glycemic index (GI) diet indicates foods that have a low GI value meaning they will take a longer time to have an affect on blood sugars and ones that have a higher value—they will act quicker to raise blood sugars. A diabetic is still going to have to use another means to decide what foods to eat though—such as the food pyramid or an exchange list as not all items on the GI diet are as healthy as they could be. Meaning a food that has a low index does not mean it is a better choice for you than some foods that are on the higher end of the scale. Using the GI diet as your sole source of meal planning is not recommended not only because the values are not indicative of the healthiest choice but also because not all foods are listed. If you are basing your diet on this method and want to add other foods that do not have GI rating you are not going to be able to properly plan. Until more information is researched on the diet or it is made more comprehensive it should be used with an approved diet for diabetics such as the exchange diet or the carbohydrate counting diet.

When you are Hungry in Between Meals

There are going to be times when you have finished your meal or snack and you are hungry again long before your next meal is scheduled or right before bed. Depending on how much time you have to go before you are supposed to eat again and what your blood sugar levels are at you may want to move your meal time up or indulge in some free food.

If this happens frequently it is time look at your eating schedule and meal plan. If you have recently added more physical activity to your daily routine, you will also have to increase your food intake to compensate for the extra energy your are using up. If this isn't the case and you are unsure why your appetite has increased or your current meal plan is no longer working, speak to your dietician to see if there are some revisions that can be made to prevent this from happening.

When you have gestational diabetes, it is recommended that you have a snack before bedtime to tide you over until the morning. It will also be important to have a bedtime snack if you are taking an insulin injection prior to bed so that your blood sugar does not become too low overnight. If neither of these scenarios applies to you, you can have some free food before bed if you are finding that you are hungry at night time. A bouillon (beef or chicken broth) might stave off hunger pangs and allow you to fall asleep.

If you are hungry at night time and your blood sugars are low, do have something to eat to raise your glucose level. If this is a frequent occurrence, you may not be eating enough food at dinner time.

Chapter IV
The Truth About Low Carb Diets

The principle of these low carb diets is to take in food low in carbohydrates so that the body is forced to use its stored fat.

By drastically reducing carbohydrates to a small fraction of a person's diet, the body goes into "ketosis". The body burns its own fat to convert into energy A person in ketosis is getting energy from ketones. Ketones are little carbon fragments that are created by the breakdown of stored fat. One feels less hungry when his or her body is in ketosis. The end result is that he or she is likely to eat less even if allowed to do so. In effect, the body is transformed from a carbohydrate-burning machine into a fat-burning one, thus making fat the primary energy source. This brings us to the most fundamental fact of dieting: the less fat you have, the lighter you weigh. The end result is the desired weight loss.

There are diets like Atkins that seem to be a dream come true. It stems from its design that a person could eat as much as he or she wants from a wide variety of food that other diets steer away from. Steaks, meat, crab, eggs, all types of protein based food are allowed since the body will burn carbohydrates first and not protein or fats. Basically, it follows the same low carb principle of reducing carbohydrate intake and forcing the body to use fat towards weight loss.

But experts are concerned about the long term safety of the diet. By contemporary medical standards, the risk of heart diseases, stroke, cancer, liver and kidney problems are very extremely high. These risks have been pointed out repeated by a number of health researches on high fat diets.

Other low carb diets are cleansing in nature such as the detox diet. It helps in the health reassessment of one's lifestyle, eating patterns and focus on foods. Here, one becomes more aware of one's food intake. However, there are individuals, such as diabetics, people with low blood sugar or eating disorders have to stay clear of it. They will find themselves more in trouble than they are already.

Low carb diets serve their purpose. But there is no substitute for the traditional, proven healthy lifestyle of a balance diet of the basic food groups in the nutritionists' pyramid order combined with the proper exercise. However, should a person still go through with these diets for whatever reason, he or she should be equipped with knowledge of not only the benefits but most especially the risks. Everyone wants that slim, healthy look.But everyone should also g o for health in a sustainable manner.

Carb Pills How to Have Carbohydrates On the Adkins or South Beach Diet

If you are trying to go on a low carbohydrate diet such as the Adkins Weight Loss Plan or the South Beach Diet and find that you have trouble reducing your carbs, you may want to try anti carb pills. These are not actually medicinal products but rather dietary supplements made from all natural ingredients not chemical blends.The reason carb smart diets such as Adkins and South Beach stay alive despite all of the negative media publicity is that they work. But, too many people find that they have trouble minimizing the amount of carbohydrates they consume for a long period of time. That is where the carb pills come in.

While more recent variations of the low carb diets have allowed more carbohydratesin the form of whole grains, it is still tempting to have a cookie from time to time. The carb pills absorb excess carbohydrates in the diet by blocking the carbohydrates consumed from being absorbed in the body.

One of the carb blocking ingredients in the pills is made from white bean extract. They are 100 percent natural and safe to consume.

It is best to take a carb blocking pill right before eating a carb heavy food or meal. They can also be taken during or after the meal, but this has a reduced effectiveness. Here is how the carb pills work on the body. Fat accumulates in the body when carbohydrates are broken down by alpha amylase, which is an enzyme produced in the pancreas. When you exert yourself through exercise or daily energy, these carbs are burned off. However, if you take in more carbs than you burn, you will store the excess as fat.Carb pills prevent the fat by preventing the excess calories from being converted through blocking the digestive enzymes from acting on them. This means that the major portion ofthe carbs are passed through the system without being absorbed.

So, do carb pills work? The scientific community has not really taken up this question because the major pharmaceutical companies fund most of the research. As the carb pills are not produced by these pharmaceutical firms, researchers have not found it worth their while to "independently" evaluate the pills. However, the companies which produce carb pills have produced their own studies. They have shown that in the short term at least, the carb blocking pills do in fact keep up to 45 grams of carbohydrates from being absorbed in the system. There may be some side effects from using the carb blocking pill. These include gastrointestinal distress, heartburn, excessive gas and diarrhea.

The two most common brands of carb pills are Carbo Lock and Ultra Carb. These pills can be expensive—a 30 day supply typically retails for $30. If you buy the products in larger quantities, you can often bring the daily cost down. If you want to have the benefits of a low carb diet but occasionally indulge in carbohydrate rich foods or meals, you might want to consider investing in carb pills which block the carbohydrates in a pasta dinner or piece of chocolate cake from turning into fat.

Protein And It's Amazing Weight Loss Power!

According to the latest statistics, the obesity epidemic continues to grow worldwide and shows no signs of stopping anytime soon. An astonishing 59.6% of Australian and New Zealand adults are overweight or obese, while 30% of Australian and New Zealand children are clinically overweight. More than half of the American population is overweight.

Those who have adequate amounts of protein in their diet, however, may find they've escaped being part of this alarming trend. That's because the latest nutritional research indicates that protein has numerous dietary benefits that give a boost to weight loss and weight management efforts. Lets look at some of the ways you can benefit from a healthy daily protein intake.

One of the principle advantages of protein is that it creates a feeling of fullness and satisfaction in the body that makes overeating much less likely. Besides being filling, protein is a smart addition to any weight loss or weight management programme because of the effect it has on carbohydrate cravings.

As nutritional research has documented, carbohydrates trigger the brain to crave more carbohydrates, leading to a cycle of carbohydrate eating that becomes hard to control. Protein can block that triggering effect in the brain. If you eat protein with a carbohydrate it will reduce the cravings caused by eating the carbohydrate.

Simply adding protein to a meal (including breakfast), provides you with an incredible advantage in your quest to lose or maintain weight. But protein provides more than just weight benefits—it provides you with an important necessity as well. Adequate daily protein intake is essential for building and maintaining lean muscle mass.

It may sound like a term that applies only to athletes, but in fact, everyone has a certain percentage of lean muscle mass in their body. The higher your percentage of lean muscle mass, the more calories you can burn in a day.

Besides determining how many calories you burn each day, lean muscle mass also serves a vital function for those trying to lose or maintain their weight. If your diet does not contain enough protein to build or maintain lean muscle mass, your body will begin to lose weight from the heart, muscle and organs.

This type of dieting is unsafe and can prove fatal. So, how much protein do you need every day? Women need approximately 80-100 grams daily, while men need roughly 120-150 grams.

But as you incorporate protein into your diet, remember that not all protein is equal when it comes to calories. For example, a serving of prime rib has 1,500 calories! That's why it is important to source your protein from healthy, lean protein sources such as fish, the white meat of chicken and turkey and very lean sources of beef. If you can see the fat…cut it off before you cook it, and don't eat it.

Ketosis Diet Low Carb Programs Activate Metabolism

Do you want to go on a Ketosis diet? Several popular diet plans are based on this principle. Adkins and South Beach are both diets which restrict carbs. This results in a ketosis diet.

The theory behind a ketosis diet is that your body will burn fat rather than carbohydrates if you deprive it of almost all carbohydrate sources. This means limiting your carb intake to just 20 grams in some cases.

Normally, the carbohydrates in food are converted into glucose. The glucose is then transported through the body and is particularly important in fuelling the brain. However, if there are very little carbs in the diet, the liver converts fat into fatty acids and ketone bodies. The ketone bodies pass into the brain and replace glucose as an energy source. Thus, the body produces ketone bodies—a state known as ketosis.

Low Carb diets take advantage of this state of ketosis. Since cells in the body can use ketones for energy instead of glucose, and since ketones are easier to produce, only a small amount of glucose is created. In other words, ketosis is the more significant process in this case. Diets low in starches and sugars do not directly affect blood sugar levels significantly, meals tend to have little direct effect on insulin levels. These diets tend to discourage insulin production in general.

Additionally, many experts argue that a ketosis diet is more like the diet our bodies have evolved to use. Prior to the advent of agriculture just a few thousand years ago, the human body had millions of years of evolution which selected for a hunter gather lifestyle. Hunter gatherers had very few carbs in their diets. They may have had the original ketosis diet.

Dr. Robert Adkins first published the Adkins Diet Revolution in 1972 which set off the modern round of low carb dieting. At the time, its appeal was limited because so many scientists and doctors condemned it. Over time, though, it gained credibility and when he republished the book as Dr. Adkins New Diet Revolution, it set off a frenzy.

Soon other ketosis diet books appeared. These included the popular South Beach diet, Zone diet, and Protein Power.

While the scientific community still hasn't acknowledged the value of the ketosis diet, they have started to make recommendations that people reduce the amount of carbohydrates in their diets. The medical community has stressed the importance of fiber in diets and recommended that children not drink juice on a regular basis.

While the popularity of ketosis diets has waned since it's height in 2004, there are still many adherents. That's because, for many people, low carb diets work when nothing else has before.

There has been much scientific research on low carb diets. There are many studies which show it works and many studies which show that it is dangerous. Because of these competing studies, advocates on both sides can pull up evidence that they are right.

Once you do your due diligence, you will be better able to decide whether to pursue a ketosis diet.

Chapter V
Detoxing

A rejuvenating 5-day body detox plan to keep you going. In the present condition, you can no longer survive a single day without encountering pollution. At work, you may not at all be so sure of the cleanliness of the water you drink or of the food you eat. When dealing with people, you can hardly get away from air pollution, be it from smokers, all sorts of sprays or from the exhaust of vehicles. This greatly affects the health in one way or another. Don't be so sure that when your body does not visibly react, it's alright. For these reasons, detoxification is necessary in order to keep a healthy body which also results to healthy mind and healthy relationship with people.

Our body has its own means of healing and detoxifying. However, when pollutants that enter our body had been accumulated more than the capacity of self cleansing, we are giving our inside mechanisms a hard time. Then the tissues are stressed and therefore lead to malfunction. And because they are weakened, the cleansing process is also affected. We definitely want a clean body. But we also need to help our system in regulating the body processes. However, you should not wait for your body organs to be stressed out and overworked before doing something. In times when the body lacks the command to keep the systems working, the person must supplement. The 5-day detox plan will do a great help

in keeping the body systems at work. The 5-day detox plan will rejuvenate the body as well as the spirit, keeping it clean and toned. Detoxification diet is a part of the 5-day detox plan. During the period of detoxification, certain foods are avoided. Your meals consist mostly of fresh fruits and green, leafy vegetables. Fats, oil, preservatives and food additives are a big no when undergoing the process of detoxification. Also, meat should be kept off because they are hard to digest. For a day or two, eating meat in any form is dropped off from the diet. Ideal foods that can be part of your diet are as follow: garlic, broccoli, beets, and beans or nuts. Only fresh fruit extracts can be taken as beverages except for grapefruit. And since water is a universal solvent, six to eight glasses of this should be recommended daily. Water is also a major factor in the detoxification process. It flushes out the toxins in the forms of perspiration, urine, or stool.

Using Herbs as Your Home Remedy for Body Detox

The accumulated toxins inside your body must be cleared in order for it to function well. Your body needs to be healed to regain energy. There is one effective way of clearing your body from these unwanted toxins and it is called body detox or body detoxification using natural herbs. However, it is not taken as a single step but a continued process so that the natural ability of your body is supported for the effective dispelling of toxins everyday. Another process being incorporated in body detox together with using herbs is limiting the toxins which enter your body. Eliminating or restricting the use of the usual culprits such as refined sugar, caffeine, alcohol, tobacco, drugs, household chemicals, and petroleum or synthetic-based body paraphernalia is a very good way of starting. You should start eating organic natural diet foods, getting regular. The following herbs that have known to be effective for many years can be used as a home remedy. These are the natural way of body detoxification.

- Psyllium seeds and husks contain high fiber which can gently act as a natural laxative. You can utilize it by soaking the seeds in water. Psyllium is generally considered as adaptogenic which supports the healthy function of your bowel. It is also useful in treating diarrhea and other irritable bowel diseases. It is a very good choice for body detoxification since its gelatinous substance after soaking absorbs toxins.

- Hydrangea root and the Joe pye weed (gravel root) helps in preventing, dissolving, and expelling stones and crystals in the bladder and kidneys. It is good to keep your kidneys free from any obstructions to stay in good working condition essential in effective elimination of toxins.

- Cascara Sagrada is used also as natural laxatives. It could be safe even for longer duration of usage where it strengthens your colon's muscles.

- Alder buckthorn's barks are also used but it must first be dried and be stored for at least one year since its fresh barks are so strong which can be considered toxic.

- Juniper berries also promote the urinary system's overall health. It detoxifies and strengthens your urinary tract, bladder, and kidneys. It is excellent for cleaning purposes but prolonged usage is not recommended because it can cause some overtaxing in your kidneys.
- Nettles also have detoxifying properties which can be extended not just in your urinary system. Nevertheless overusing it can display similar effects as the juniper berries.
- Burdock seeds and roots are similar to nettles. It has mild and cleansing diuretic action but has stronger effects. Heavy metals inside your body can be removed by using burdock.
- Basil, cypress, celery, grapefruit, lemon, fennel, rosemary, thyme, and patchouli contains essential oils effective for flushing out toxins underneath your skin and stimulating circulation of your lymph.
- Dandelion root and milk thistle help in cleansing and strengthening your liver. Milk thistle has silymarin which does not only protect your liver but helps in regenerating itself. Dandelion root helps in removing waste products from your gallbladder and kidneys. You would never have any problems if your body needs detoxification at home. You can try using these wonderful herbs to obtain their natural remedies. Rejuvenate yourself and feel good about it.

When to Say That Detox Diet Guide on Cleansing Your Body Is Safe

A detox diet may sound very reassuring for it is a fact that toxics are bad for the health of a person. These diets however encourage you to eat foods that are natural which involves lots of veggies and water. Well, you can also add all the stuff that is good for your body. You could even hear news about celebrities having detox diets as well as those people who are subjected to alcohol or drug rehabs and are detoxifying themselves. So, you would really ask if detox diets are safe.

The answer is dependent on who is going to utilize such type of diet. Detox diets like many fad diets can later on display side effects that are harmful especially for teenagers. To avoid misconception, you need to understand the lingo. Toxins are poisons or chemicals that have harmful side effects on your body. It could come from water or food, chemicals used for growing or preparing food, and from the air that you breathe. These toxins are processed in kidneys and liver eliminating it in the forms of urine, feces, and sweat. Most people who are supporting detox diets are saying that dehydration or emotional stress is the cause why toxins do not leave the body properly during wastes elimination. Instead, these toxins are just hanging around the digestive system, gastrointestinal systems, lymph, skin, and hair. Even detox diet's proponents said that these toxins are the promoters of problems such as headaches, tiredness, acne, and nausea. So you must understand that basic idea behind a detox diet is to give up temporarily the foods that are known to have toxins. It is a means of purifying and purging your body from all bad stuff. Detox diets may also vary however most of it is involved in several versions of displaying fast results. You need to give up foods within a few days, then after that, gradually reintroducing a particular food in your diet. Lots of detox diets also encourages you to go through colonic irrigation or enema to clean up your colon. The enema washes out your colon and rectum using water. But then others still recommend taking herbal supplements during the purification procedure. There lots of available detox diets anywhere. Typically, it involves one or two days of complete liquid diet. For the succeeding four to five days, add brown rice, steamed vegetables, and fruit that are all organic to your diet is advised. After one week of eating these foods, you will then gradually introduce certain foods except for wheat, red meat, eggs, sugar, and junk food in your diet.

People who are having their detox diets are advised to chew up their foods thoroughly, drink only very little amount of water while eating, and relax before eating. It is much better if you add one glass of lemon juice in every meal. There can be numerous claims made about the effects of detox diets on a person. It can prevent and cure diseases to give you extra energy so that you stay clear-headed and focused. Well, anyone who prefers low-fat but high fiber diets will probably feel much better and more healthy. But no matter what good things detox diets proponents said, still it is up to you to decide whether to try it or not for your own safety. It is because there is no scientific evidence that these diets get rid of body toxins faster or if the elimination of it can make you more healthy and energetic.

All natural body detox for body cleansing and total mind rejuvenation When we hear the word toxin, we mistakenly think of poison in a labeled bottled. Indeed, toxins are poisonous, but they are not necessarily labeled when they enter our body in many and perhaps unthinkable ways. Imagine how minute and invisible microbes are and that they can penetrate into our pores. And everyday exposure to street life allows you to meet all sorts of air pollution. If germs can enter your body through very small openings, how much more to total exposure where viruses can easily enter? So what happens when the body is overloaded with pollutants? Well, it's not as simple as just getting sick. Mind processing is significantly affected and all the rest of your body. Pollutants block or slow down the delivery of needed nutrients and oxygen to all parts of the body. And since the brain is the major consumer of oxygen, it has the tendency to be damaged. Have you noticed that after doing a hard-hitting mental work, you feel very exhausted even when you were just seated for hours?

It is because the brain can sometimes override the whole body. So when there are lots of toxins in you, your mind becomes sluggish too. And most of the time, it's tough to protect ourselves to the extent of being disease-proof. Although the body provides its own system of healing, we need to take care of it and help it function better. That is why we need to detoxify. Detoxification helps in rejuvenation of the mind as much as it cleanses the body. The safest way to detoxify is having it the natural way—through proper diet. In this process of cleansing, you reduce your intake of junk. This means that you must avoid products that obstruct your filtering system.

These products are fats, alcohol, caffeine, and food additives. While you stay away from these foods, you replace them with easy to digest fruits and vegetables. They are not only rich in vitamins, but they supplement the body with energy boosting nutrients. Surely, they are clean, given that they are prepared freshly and cleanly. The fibers in fruits and vegetables toss the toxins out. In detoxification, fasting for a short period of time will catalyze the process. Of course this should be done under the supervision of your nutritionist or doctor. During the process, solid foods are avoided. Your intake is solely made of fruit juice and herbal teas. Researches are made to prove that fasting decreases the stress on the digestive system. By emptying the stomach, toxins are also flushed out of the body. And the liquids that you take keep you away from starving. Nevertheless, fasting is quite critical so it is advised that a physician must be consulted first. Preferably, fast during the weekends when your time is allotted merely to relaxation. In addition to fruit juices, some supplements are recommended for safety. To name a few are the fermented soybeans and algae powder. Fermented soy beans support the colon function and help produce the good intestinal bacteria which are major proponents of the inner cleansing process. In parallel, the algae powder gives you the feeling of being full. It supplies ample protein to ease the fatigue that some people experience during fasting. Detoxification in the whole is a matter of a good system of living.

Body Detox Herbs Can Do Wonder in Your Lives

It is a fact that some pesticides, chemicals, and certain fumes are present in the environment that is affecting your immune system and jeopardizing your health. Moreover, the foods that you eat can lead to a toxic atmosphere lowering your overall immunity. Toxic load is the condition of tissues and cells where internal terrain is developed after food consumption of highly processed foods. Your body needs to be cleansed from these unwanted toxins. The process is called detoxification.

Although you have the kidney and liver which are organs considered as natural detoxifiers filtering out the impurities of the bodies, you need to consider other ways to detoxify your body from toxins. Some of the methods can be extreme like long fasting from juice drinks or dialysis.

Take note, your immune system is the defense mechanism of your body. So, disease and infections should be prevented before it affects your whole body through toxin's removal. As you could observe, the illness' frequency of a person is dependent on the immune's system strength which is composed of complex networks of nodes and lymph channels.

There are detox herbs that are beneficial in making your immune system strong. These herbs are the perfect and natural way of removing toxins from your immune systems to minimize acquired illnesses and to develop your general well-being.

Several herbs for detoxifying are much better for improving your immune systems than others. However, there are specific considerations for the detoxification program that you choose. But the following detox herbs can be used according to your needs.

- **Carrot tops (*Daucus carota*)** Carrot tops are an under-appreciated source of relief for all sorts of urinary tract problems and symptoms. The Amish swear by it, dedicating significant acreage to carrots just for this reason. Carrot Top Tea can clear up skin blemishes, flush the kidneys and bladder, and clean the blood of toxins. Carrot tops are also helpful in clearing the kidneys and urinary tract (as well as the prostate). They are also highly alkalizing to the blood, taking stress off the kidneys.

- **Goldenrod (*Solidago virguarea*)** Goldenrod is used as an aquaretic agent, meaning that it promotes the loss of water from the body (as compared to a diuretic, which promotes the loss of both water and electrolytes such as salt). It is used frequently in Europe to treat urinary tract inflammation and to prevent or treat kidney stones. In fact, goldenrod has received official recognition in Germany for its effectiveness in getting rid of kidney stones, and it is commonly found in teas to help "flush out" kidney stones and stop inflammatory diseases of the urinary tract. Goldenrod is said to wash out bacteria and kidney stones by increasing the flow of urine, and also, soothe inflamed tissues and calm muscle spasms in the urinary tract.

People would really need to detoxify themselves due to the presence of toxins in processed foods and in polluted air. Using herbs is not new in detoxification programs because its cleansing and healing properties have been known for so many years. Thus, it is now being accepted in the detoxification concept treating patients worldwide.

These herbs can effectively flush out unwanted toxins from your immune system allowing you to look and feel great. It can save you from acquiring severe illnesses like diabetes Brilliant detox herbs can really do wonders in a person's life.

Chapter VI
Nutritional Supplements

Why take a vitamin?

Despite the fact that people are living hectic lifestyles more than ever, they are following a more healthy diet and exercising on a regular basis. You might wonder if the recommendation by the health industry to take a multivitamin every day is still valid in light of the trend of people becoming healthier. If you are eating a variety of foods, there's a good chance you are getting the vitamins and minerals your body needs to perform routine functions to keep your body healthy. However, you're not completely out of the woods.

When you use heat to cook your food (grill, fry, bake), the heating process removes some of your food's beneficial nutrients. In addition, if you are plagued with stress or you if you are taking medication there's a chance that you are losing a significant amount of vitamins and minerals that you consume. Taking vitamins on a regular basis can increase your chances of getting all the nutrients your body needs.

The benefits of taking vitamins go beyond meeting the recommended dietary allowances. How healthy you are depends on more than just diet and the amount of exercise you obtain. There are other outside factors that can predispose you to develop certain health issues. For example, how much of a risk you have for developing cancer of heart disease is largely dependent upon whether or not others in your family developed these conditions. For sometime it was believed that an individual had very little recourse in these situations. Studies conducted by Harvard University researchers revealed that taking a multivitamin every day can reduce an individual's risk to develop these conditions.

To determine your specific needs, you should visit your doctor for a complete evaluation of your dietary needs. Your doctor will be able to recommend the type of vitamins that are best for you. It may very well be the case that a common multivitamin is all that you need. If this is the case, you can visit any nutrition center or grocery store and find aisles of multivitamins.

Pharmaceutical Grade Vitamins vs. Regular Vitamins

Vitamins are necessary for human life and health. They are required in minute amounts, and with the exception of Vitamin B12, cannot be manufactured in your bodies. These organic compounds need to be obtained from diet, and if deprived of a particular vitamin, you will suffer from disease specific to that vitamin. It is a matter of record that you are not getting enough vitamins. Though we Americans are living longer, our quality of life leaves much to be desired.

The thirteen different vitamins are classified into two main categories:

- Water Soluble Vitamins—They dissolve easily in water. They are Vitamin C and the eight types of Vitamins B, B-1, B-2, B-3, B-5, B-6, B-7, B-9, and B-12.
- Fat Soluble Vitamins—With the help of lipids, they are absorbed through the intestinal tract. These vitamins are Vitamins A. D, E, and K.

The term Vitamin does not mean to include essential nutrients, such as, dietary minerals, essential fatty acids, or essential amino acids; neither does it mean to include other nutrients that just promote health, and may not be essential.

The Different Grades of Vitamins

Vitamin supplements are taken by more than 75% of the world's population. With the plethora of different brands, it becomes difficult to know what is what. Vitamins and other nutritional supplements are made from three different grades of raw materials:

Pharmaceutical Grade—It meets pharmaceutical standards
- Food Grade—It meets standards for human consumption
- Feed Grade—It meets standards for animal consumption

The main difference is of quality and purity. Due to the addition of various other substances, no product is 100% pure. Pharmaceutical Grade Vitamins must be in excess of 99% purity containing no binders, fillers, excipients—substances used as diluents for a drug—dyes, or unknown substances. Regular Vitamins of the other two grades are available as Over The Counter (OTC) products, whereas pharmaceutical grade vitamins are only available through prescriptions.

Pharmaceutical grade vitamins are formulated to yield a higher degree of bioavailability—the degree at which the vitamin is absorbed into a living system. As these vitamins can be absorbed into your body quickly, they improve and enhance the quality of your life rapidly.

Of late, the American vitamin industry has gained a lot of bad reputation, and many feel it is rightly deserved. People walk into stores and pharmacies to buy regular vitamins. In some of the cases, the ingredients specified on the label are not in conformity with what they find inside the bottle. A variety of ingredients do not absorb into the body.

More and more people are opting for pharmaceutical grade vitamins, as they are available through prescriptions from doctors and licensed medical practitioners. Pharmaceutical grade vitamins, vis-à-vis regular vitamins, have been tested for their quality and ability to give results. They are tested by third parties to confirm that the bottles contain what they profess to contain.

Probiotics & Their Use As A Dietary Supplement

Many people are unfamiliar with probiotics, but there are studies to show that these supplements may be beneficial in the treatment of various ailments. Probiotics are dietary supplements that contain possible beneficial bacteria. Certain types of yogurt, for example, contain probiotics in therapeutic quantities. This simply means that some foods contain enough of this supplement to be helpful and is measured in quantities where it cannot be overindulged.

Many people are unfamiliar with probiotics, but there are studies to show that these supplements may be beneficial in the treatment of various ailments. Probiotics are dietary supplements that contain possible beneficial bacteria. Certain types of yogurt, for example, contain probiotics in therapeutic quantities. This simply means that some foods contain enough of this supplement to be helpful and is measured in quantities where it cannot be overindulged.

Probiotics are believed to assist the body's digestive system and are sometimes recommended by physicians. More frequently, however, probiotics are recommended by nutritionists as part of a healthy, well balanced diet program. Some theories even exist that suggest these dietary supplements may help to strengthen the immune system. While there is no recorded evidence to suggest that probiotics can replace damaged parts of the body's digestive tracts, there is proof that it can form temporary associations that may help to produce the same functions while the damaged areas have additional time to recover. By allowing the body with additional recovery time, probiotics may offer both valuable and temporary assistance.

In addition to aiding in digestion and improving the immune system, probiotics are also thought to help prevent constipation, reduce the occurrence of insomnia and may help to reduce stress-related ailments. Stress is believed to be responsible for the onset of many illnesses, which is why research continues in an attempt to find ways to help reduce these ailments. What is one of the main illnesses related to stress? The answer is high blood pressure which, alone, can be extremely dangerous and may lead to other problems if not maintained.

Certain types of commercial products, namely health foods, contain a specific amount of probiotics. As mentioned previously in this article, such products may include yogurt or sauerkraut. Probiotic foods and dietary products are the most common forms of the dietary supplements, but tablets and capsules are also sometimes made available. Individuals may ask their physician about various types of foods and the amount of probiotics that each contains.

This is to be used for informational purposes only and is not intended to be used as professional medical advice. The information contained herein should not be used in place of, or in conjunction with, a doctor's recommendation . Prior to beginning any treatment regimen, including one that involves the use of probiotics, an individual who develops an illness of any type should consult a licensed physician for proper diagnosis and treatment.

Resveratrol Capsules—Tiny Ounces of Health!

In an effort to discover the therapeutic effects of diverse plants, scientists have started to isolate different substances thought to be benefic. One of the examples that can be given is represented by Polygonum Cuspidatum, from which Resveratrol (3, 5, 4'- trihydroxystilbene) was isolated and taken for extensive research. Today, that substance is known extremely well and it appears to be more beneficial than anyone could ever imagine. Available over the Internet, Resveratrol is a constitutive element of red wine and in studies, has shown that one of its most powerful effects is the protection offered for the cardiovascular system.

From the moment when it was isolated and up to the present time, many discoveries have been made about Resveratrol and its effects. Studies have been performed on mice and the findings were more than satisfactory. It seems that a high Resveratrol dose has amazing effects, not only cardio protective but also inhibits tumor growth (Resveratrol supplements have been considered for their chemo preventive action in studies) and even increases the lifespan of lab rats. All these effects have been observed in the studies made on Resveratrol molecule, and has been made available now on the Internet in the form of health supplements.

As everyone knows, a large percent of the studies made on mice have provided answers to treatments that can be performed or given to humans. Resveratrol capsules contain a high dosage of Trans-Resveratrol that may offer all the effects presented above and even some that are still being studied. The Resveratrol molecule is known to reduce inflammation caused by immune mechanisms in affections such as psoriasis and Chron's disease, representing much more effective alternatives than other options considered. Also, the same Trans-Resveratrol in the herbal capsules is known to reduce the stress levels in rodents and thus, protect the organism from further disease.

If you are interested in Resveratrol, make sure that you read some of the conclusions presented by the studies made and also what the recommended doses compare against those doses given in studies. Don't be scared if the doses recommended are high as they need to be that way in order for the substance to be as efficient as possible. Try the 1000 mg Resveratrol capsule with Trans-Resveratrol from natural herbs and you will definitely be impressed with the results. They represent exactly the kind of new dietary health supplements that can positively produce results. In studies, Resveratrol shows that it protects the heart but also your circulatory system, reducing the risk of vascular attack. It is a well known fact that much of the ischemic and vascular attacks are caused by increased stress. Resveratrol allows the body to respond better to stress even though the mechanisms by which this substance acts have not been completely elucidated.

As a final conclusion, there are three things one must understand about First, it appears to require higher doses than one can get from wine in order to have improved beneficial effects. Second, it is 100% safe and in studies, has an effect on a wide variety of illnesses (inflammatory, cancerous and age-related such as Alzheimer). Last, but not least it represents a natural herbal supplement, which is an incredible natural advantage over a hard drug. It can be taken by those interested in dietary regimes, in capsules of 500 or 300 mg. Just make sure that you do not give Resveratrol supplements to children under the age of 18, as the studies on child development are still not conclusive. Other from that, feel free to take advantage of all the potentially amazing benefits brought on by the Resveratrol herbal capsules!

Best Vitamin Supplements

Most people want to improve their health, particularly if they can do it easily. Since the way modern food is processed can destroy nutrients, many people choose to supplement their diets by taking vitamin pills. What are the best vitamin supplements to maximize health? Here is a suggested list.

Always consult your physician before you start taking vitamins. Your medical advisor is the only person who can determine what the best vitamin supplements and dosages are for you.

The basics

A multivitamin tablet is a great foundation when looking for the best vitamin supplements. It will contain some of all the basic vitamins and minerals you need and in some cases, a full dose. For example, the amount of Vitamin A in multivitamins is plenty and a separate Vitamin A tablet won't be needed.

Vitamin B complex, which includes 11 different B vitamins, contributes to the health of the nervous system. It is beneficial for medication overuse, alcoholism or recovery from a serious illness. B vitamins assist in reducing the effects of stress and support the adrenal glands. They aid in the metabolism of carbohydrates, fats and proteins and are essential for the health of your skin, hair, eyes, mouth and liver.

Vitamin B-3 is also known as niacin or niacinamide. It helps maintain healthy functioning of the nervous system, digestive system and skin.

Vitamin B-6 combats carpal tunnel syndrome, joint pain, trigger finger, sensitivity to bright light, burning or tingling in the extremities and inability to recall dreams. It works in combination with magnesium and zinc.

Vitamin B-12 is used as a tonic. It assists in the conversion of iron to hemoglobin in the blood, helps normalize hormone production and increases short-term memory in the elderly. It also contributes to nervous system health.

Folic acid is an essential B vitamin that promotes heart health. Pregnant women need ample supplies of folic acid to reduce the risk of serious birth defects in their babies.

Vitamin C is a strong antioxidant. It reacts with free radicals in the bloodstream to combat cell damage, so it can be considered a cancer fighter. It is important in immune system health and collagen formation. Some people believe high doses of vitamin C can help fight colds, but research to support this is mixed. It is present in citrus fruit and prevents scurvy, a disease caused by vitamin C deficiency.

Vitamin D helps promote healthy bones, largely by helping the body absorb calcium. Vitamin D can reduce the risk of diabetes, heart attack, muscle and bone pain, rheumatoid arthritis, multiple sclerosis, and cancers of the breast, colon, prostate, ovaries, esophagus and lymphatic system. It may also help lower blood pressure. It stimulates the pancreas to make insulin and regulates the immune system.

Vitamin E is a fat-soluble vitamin that fights free radicals whose accumulation can lead to premature cell aging. In addition, vitamin E enhances immune response, which is beneficial in preventing and fighting cancer. Studies suggest it may reduce the risk of prostate cancer. It was formerly believed that Vitamin E helped reduce the risk of heart attack, but recent studies suggest it may increase that risk.

Calcium is necessary for bone maintenance and assists in muscle contraction and nerve function. It may also help prevent colon cancer.

Magnesium works with calcium to build bones. It helps keep muscles strong and nerves alert, as well as helping protect the heart from the stress of exercise. It may also protect against type two diabetes.

Optional extras

Beta carotene supplements the activity of vitamin A. It is a powerful antioxidant and immune system enhancer.

Chromium picolinate stabilizes blood sugar and may promote weight loss as part of a balanced diet and exercise regimen. It can also be used for body building, decreased and increased blood sugar levels and morning sickness.

Coenzyme Q10 is a major antioxidant used in the transfer of cellular respiration inside the inner mitochondrial membranes of the body's cells. It supports heart health.

Lutein promotes eye health. It may protect against aging related eye diseases, including macular degeneration and cataracts.

Selenium binds with heavy metals and helps the body get rid of them. It supports the immune system and may protect against some forms of cancer.

Zinc is another antioxidant supplement believed to be helpful in shortening the duration of colds. People with zinc deficiency may have significantly higher glucose levels and lower insulin levels than similar patients without normal zinc levels.

If you are experiencing health problems, do some research on the Internet to find what the best vitamin supplements are for your condition. People who prefer to avoid taking prescription drugs may be able to find solutions by selecting the best vitamin supplements supported by research studies.

Why should you take Vitamin B?

1. Vitamin B1 (Thiamine) that is found in bread, pork, and whole bread. It helps with digestion, growth, and it keeps the nerves healthy.

2. Vitamin B2 (riboflavin) which is very important for the body to produce red blood cells that is found in red meat, mushrooms, milk, etc.

3. Vitamin B3 (Niacin) which is essential in converting the food or supplements into energy. It aids the digestive system, skin, and nerves so that they will function normally.

4. Vitamin B6 (Pyridoxine) that plays essential role in maintaining the body's red blood cells. It is also important in producing antibodies and nerve tissues.

5. Vitamin B9 (Folic acid) which is found in fresh fruits, green plants, yeast, and liver. It is important for the division and growth of cells.

6. Vitamin B12 (Pantothenic acid) which is essential for the body to release energy from proteins, fats, and carbohydrates. It also plays an important role in developing the central nervous system and cell building.

There are many reasons why people should take Vitamin B and these are the following:

1. Vitamin B1 also known as Thiamine is considered the most important type of vitamin B today. It is anti-neuritic and anti-beriberi. It also promotes growth, stimulates brain action, and safeguards the muscles that protect the heart. Without it, the nervous system will not function well. Thiamine maintains red blood count, promotes healthy skin, and improves circulation. Its benefits also include protection against lead poisoning and prevention of fluid retention that is connected with heart diseases.

Thiamine sources

To avoid Vitamin B1 deficiency, include wholegrain cereals, oats, and rice to the diet. Also, grab some pineapples, pork, and nuts to maintain the supply of Thiamine.

2. Vitamin B2 or riboflavin is essential in formation of antibodies and red blood cells. Without it, pregnant women may risk the health of the developing fetus. In addition, riboflavin is important in maintaining good vision and building tissue.

Riboflavin sources

To keep the fetus healthy and maintain good eyesight, eat some dairy products, fish, broccoli, asparagus, lean meats, spinach, and poultry.

3. Vitamin B3 or Niacin is also important in converting fat, carbohydrates, and proteins into energy. It also aids the digestive system to function normally and it promotes healthy nerves and skin. Niacin deficiency can lead to lose of appetite, muscular weakness, skin problems, and indigestion.

Niacin sources

To keep energized and healthy, eat beef liver, tuna, sardines, cereals, lambs, sardines, etc.

4. Vitamin B6 or Pyridoxine keeps the nervous and immune systems healthy. It also fights known heart diseases, maintains normal hormone production, and most importantly, it keep the red blood cells from becoming dangerous blood clots.

Pyridoxine sources

Keep the heart healthy by eating fortified cereals, poultry, some vegetables and fruits, soybeans, wheat germ, and fish.

5. Vitamin B9 or Folic acid has attracted more attention when it was proven essential for pregnant women. It assures healthy fetus by keeping it away from neural tube defects. In addition, it also keeps the heart healthy by lowering homocysteine levels.

Folic acid sources

Have a healthy baby and heart by just eating grains, meat, beans, vegetables, fruits, and dairy products.

6. Vitamin B12 or Pantothenic acid is very important for reproduction, growth, and normal physiological function. Vitamin B12 deficiency can lead to retardation, functional impairments, and sudden death.

Pantothenic sources

Stay healthy by eating sweet potato, mushroom, yogurt, avocado, lobsters, and organ meats.

Vitamin B is very important for the body to function well. Knowing its benefit can improve health or even save lives.

Your Digestion

The human body's digestion is ONLY as efficient as the stomach's ability to begin the process. To be healthy, your system has to assimilate food, distribute the nutrients, and eliminate waste through the bowels. 80% of our body's energy is expended by the digestive process.

Because our entire system functions through enzymes, we must supplement our enzymes. Aging deprives us of our ability to produce necessary enzymes. So does stress, emotions, illness/disease. Our lives are dependent on these enzymes. Natural supplemental enzymes are de-rived from plant foods and are known as plant enzymes.

Supplemental plant enzymes come in a capsule form and are swallowed WITH food to assist in the digestion of that particular meal/snack. They work throughout the entire digestive system, from the esophagus to the rectum. Because of their ability to aid in digestion throughout our entire digestive process as well as support the endocrine system, plant enzymes are the most useful to the human body.

It is important to remember that poorly digested car-bohydrates will ferment in the intestinal tract. Poorly di-gested fats turn rancid, and proteins putrefy in your system if undigested.

Protease is active in a wide range of pH's, ensuring that proper protein digestion will initiate in the stomach. Protease enzymes are necessary for the complete hydro-lysis of proteins thus liberating amino acids, the building blocks for every cell in our body including muscle, tissue, blood cells and immune cells. Oral supplementation with L. acidophilus can enhance the body's anti-infective mecha-nisms of defense

Our glucose balance is the most precious and high-precision balance in the body. The brain needs 140 grams (0.3 lbs) of glucose, or we will get a headache. We need an additional 40 (0.09 lbs) grams to make red blood cells.

Yet, we ingest at least 1000 grams (2.2 lbs) of sugar or more each day. How does our body handle the surplus?

We produce more insulin, which carries glucose to our cells. Enzymes can make a big difference. Amylase and sucrose work well in the breakdown of sugar and help with gaining control of how much we ingest. Protease provides a nontoxic environment. This is one way to start the "clean-up" process and maintain the end result.

The broad spectrum of stable and functional digestive enzymes addresses this concern.

Start taking magnesium and chromium rich diets to control your diabetes

Manganese—Manganese is vital in the production of natural insulin and therefore important in the treatment of diabetes. It is found in citrus fruits, in the outer covering of nuts, grains and in the green leaves of edible plants.

The loss of magnesium in diabetic ketosis has been known for many years. About 37 percent of infants born to diabetic mothers have been found to be lacking in this mineral. It has also been found that children aged five to 18 years with well-controlled type-1 diabetes have lows serum magnesium values.

Magnesium—Magnesium also decreases the need for vitamin B6 and if it is increased in the diet, the amount of xanthurenic acid in the blood is reduced, even without vitamin B6 supplement. Moreover, magnesium is also necessary to active enzymes containing vitamin B6. Blood magnesium being particularly low in diabetic, it may be reasonably inferred that diabetes can result from a combined deficiency of vitamin B6 and magnesium. It may therefore, be advisable for any person with diabetes or a family history of the disease to take the at least 500 mg of magnesium and 10 mg of B6 daily.

Magnesium is widely distributed in foods. It forms part of the chlorophyll in green leaves. Other good sources of this mineral are nuts, Soya bean, alfalfa, apple, fig, lemon, peach, almond, whole grains, brown rice, sunflower seeds and sesame seeds.

Chromium—According to Dr. Richard A. Anderson, at the U. S. Department of Agriculture's Human Nutrition Research Center in Beltsville, Maryland, whatever the blood sugar problem, chromium tends to normalize it. Dr. Anderson believes that increased prevalence of type-2 diabetes is partly due to a deficiency of chromium in the diet.

Chromium has been found beneficial in the prevention and treatment of diabetes. Columbia University scientists, in a study reported in the American Journal of Clinical Nutrition established chromium's benefits for type-2 diabetes. They confirmed that chromium enhances insulin production in the body. Some other researchers have also confirmed that chromium helps stabilize blood sugar and increases energy.

Studies have also revealed that chromium supplements control total cholesterol and triglyceride levels and raise the good or HDL cholesterol. In some patients with impaired glucose tolerance, especially children with protein malnutrition, glucose tolerance showed improvement after they were given chromium supplements.

The recommended daily allowance of chromium is 50 to 100 micrograms. Some foods rich in chromium, besides broccoli, are whole grain cereals, nuts, mushrooms, rhubarb, Bengal gram, kidney beans, Soya beans, black gram, betel leaves, bottle gourd, corn oil, brewer's yeast, pomegranate and pineapple.

Chapter VII
Diabetes Recipes

Beef or Turkey Stew

This dish goes nicely with a green leaf lettuce and cucumber salad and a dinner roll. Plantains or corn can be used in place of the potatoes.

Ingredients:
1 pound lean beef or turkey breast, cut into cubes
2 Tbsp. whole wheat flour
¼ tsp. salt (optional)
¼ tsp. pepper
¼ tsp. cumin
1½ Tbsp. olive oil
2 cloves garlic, minced
2 medium onions, sliced
2 stalks celery, sliced
1 medium red/green bell pepper, sliced
1 medium tomato, finely minced
5 cups beef or turkey broth, fat removed
5 small potatoes, peeled and cubed
12 small carrots, cut into large chunks
1¼ cups green peas

Directions:

Preheat oven to 375 °F.

Mix the whole wheat flour with salt, pepper, and cumin. Roll the beef or turkey cubes in the mixture. Shake off excess flour.

In a large skillet, heat olive oil over medium-high heat. Add beef or turkey cubes and sauté until nicely brown, about 7–10 minutes

Place beef or turkey in an ovenproof casserole dish.

Add minced garlic, onions, celery, and peppers to skillet and cook until vegetables are tender, about 5 minutes.

Stir in tomato and broth. Bring t o a boil and pour over turkey or beef in casserole dish. Cover dish tightly and bake f or I h our a t 3 75 ° F.

Remove from oven and stir in potatoes, carrots, and peas. Bake for another 20–25 minutes or until tendeVI

Beef or Turkey Stew

This dish goes nicely with a green leaf lettuce and cucumber salad and a dinner roll. Plantains or corn can be used in place of the potatoes.

Ingredients:
1 pound lean beef or turkey breast, cut into cubes
2 Tbsp. whole wheat flour
¼ tsp. salt (optional)
¼ tsp. pepper
¼ tsp. cumin
1½ Tbsp. olive oil
2 cloves garlic, minced
2 medium onions, sliced
2 stalks celery, sliced
1 medium red/green bell pepper, sliced
1 medium tomato, finely minced
5 cups beef or turkey broth, fat removed
5 small potatoes, peeled and cubed
12 small carrots, cut into large chunks
1¼ cups green peas

Directions:

Preheat oven to 375 °F.

Mix the whole wheat flour with salt, pepper, and cumin. Roll the beef or turkey cubes in the mixture. Shake off excess flour.

In a large skillet, heat olive oil over medium-high heat. Add beef or turkey cubes and sauté until nicely brown, about 7–10 minutes

Place beef or turkey in an ovenproof casserole dish.

Add minced garlic, onions, celery, and peppers to skillet and cook until vegetables are tender, about 5 minutes.

Stir in tomato and broth. Bring t o a boil and pour over turkey or beef in casserole dish. Cover dish tightly and bake f or 1 h our a t 3 75 ° F.

Remove from oven and stir in potatoes, carrots, and peas. Bake for another 20–25 minutes or until tender.

Caribbean Red Snapper

This fish can be served on top of vegetables along with whole grain rice and garnished with parsley. Salmon or chicken breast can be used in place of red snapper.

Ingredients:
2 Tbsp. olive oil
1 medium onion, chopped
½ cup red pepper, chopped
½ cup carrots, cut into strips
1 clove garlic, minced
½ cup dry white wine
¾ pound red snapper fillet
1 large tomato, chopped
2 Tbsp. pitted ripe olives, chopped
2 Tbsp. crumbled low-fat feta or low-fat ricotta cheese

Directions:

In a large skillet, heat olive oil over medium heat. Add onion, red pepper, carrots, and garlic. Sauté mixture for 10 minutes. Add wine and bring to boil. Push vegetables to one side of the pan.

Arrange fillets in a single layer in center of skillet. Cover and cook for 5 minutes.

Add tomato and olives. Top with cheese. Cover and cook for 3 minutes or until fish is firm but moist.

Transfer fish to serving platter. Garnish with vegetables and pan juices.

Chunky Apple Cake
1 c. all-purpose flour
½ tsp. ground nutmeg
½ tsp. ground cinnamon
¼ tsp. salt
3/4 c. granulated sugar
3 Tbsp. stick margarine, softened
1 egg
2 Tbsp. low-fat milk (1%)
2 large baking apples, cored and sliced (3 cups)
1 tsp. granulated sugar
½ tsp. ground cinnamon
Exchanges: 1 ½ carbohydrates
½ fat

1. Pre-heat the oven to 350 degrees. Spray an 8x8x2 baking pan with nonstick cooking spray.
2. In a medium bowl, whisk together the flour, nutmeg, cinnamon and salt.
3. In another medium bowl, with an electric mixer at medium speed, beat the sugar and the margarine together until fluffy (about 2 minutes). Beat in the egg and milk until smooth, about 1 minutes. Add the flour mixture to the margarine mixture in thirds, beating until smooth, (about 2 minutes). With a large spoon, stir in the apples until evenly distributed. Spread the batter in the prepared pan.
    4. In a small bowl combine the sugar and cinnamon for the topping, then sprinkle evenly on the batter. Bake until brown and the sides start to pull away from the sides of the pan, approximately 40-45 minutes.

Collard Greens
1 large bunch of collard greens (64 oz. cut and washed)
3 c. low-sodium chicken broth or homemade chicken stock without meat
2 medium onions, chopped
3 whole garlic cloves, crushed
1 tsp. red pepper flakes
1 tsp. black pepper
Exchanges: 2 vegetables
1. Wash and cut greens.
2. Mix greens in large stock pot together with the remaining ingredients.
3. Cook until tender. (Allow flavors to blend by preparing the dish early in the day. The longer it blends the better it tastes!)

Fresh Salsa
3 lg. tomatoes, peeled and diced
½ c. white onion, chopped fine
½ jalapeno pepper, chopped
1 Anaheim pepper, seeded and chopped
½ sweet red pepper, chopped
2 tbsp. cilantro, chopped
¼ tsp. salt
fresh juice from ½ lime
1 tsp. white wine vinegar
1 tbsp. water or tomato juice
Exchanges: 2 vegetables
1. Place tomatoes in a colander to reduce the tomato liquid while you prepare the rest of the ingredients. Place a bowl under the colander if you want to collect the tomato juice.
2. Put all ingredients in a glass, ceramic or stainless steel bowl. Mix well , let stand for 30 minutes.
3. Serve salsa with baked tortillas, with meats, or with other main dishes.

Grilled Shrimp with Pasta and Pineapple Salsa
2 15 oz. cans of pineapple chunks, packed in their own juice, drained
1 large red pepper, chopped
1 large red onion, chopped
1 jalapeno pepper, minced
½ c. orange juice
1/3 c. lime juice
1 ½ lb. large shrimp, peeled and deveined
6 cups cooked rotini pasta
Exchanges: 3½ starch

3 very lean meat

1. In a large bowl, combine all the salsa ingredients EXCEPT the shrimp and the pasta.

2. Prepare an outside grill with an oiled rack set 4 inches above the heat source. On a gas grill set the heat to high.

3. Grill the shrimp on each side for 2 minutes.

4. Toss the pasta with the salsa, arrange the shrimp on top and serve.

Oven Fried Chicken

3 lbs. whole fryer chicken, cut-up

1 c. skim milk

1 tsp. thyme

1 tsp. garlic powder

1 tsp. onion powder

1 tsp. parsley flakes

1 tsp. paprika

1 tsp. black pepper

1 tsp. salt

1/8 tsp. red pepper flakes

1 c. flour

Exchanges: 1½ starch

4 lean meat

5½ fat

1. Pre-heat oven to 450 degrees. Skin chicken and place in the milk.

2. In a separate bowl, place all the seasonings into the flour and mix.

3. Dredge chicken parts into flour, making sure all pieces are well coated, place on pan sprayed with non-stick cooking spray. After placing chicken on pan, spray top of chicken with non-stick cooking spray.

4. Place in oven for 45 minutes until juices run clear.

Rice with Chicken, Spanish Style

This is a good way to get vegetables into the meal plan. Serve with a mixed green salad and some whole wheat bread.

Ingredients:
2 Tbsp. olive oil
2 medium onions, chopped
6 cloves garlic, minced
2 stalks celery, diced
2 medium red/green peppers, cut into strips
1 cup mushrooms, chopped
2 cups uncooked wholegrain rice
3 pounds boneless chicken breast, cut into bite-sized pieces, skin removed
1½ tsp. salt (optional)
2½ cups low-fat chicken broth
Saffron or SazónTM for color
3 medium tomatoes, chopped
1 cup frozen peas
1 cup frozen corn
1 cup frozen green beans
Olives or capers for garnish (optional)

Directions:

Heat olive oil over medium heat in a non-stick pot. Add onion, garlic, celery, red/green pepper, and mushrooms. Cook over medium heat, stirring often, for 3 minutes or until tender.

Add whole grain rice and sauté for 2–3 minutes, stirring constantly to mix all ingredients.

Add chicken, salt, chicken broth, water, Saffron/ SazónTM, and tomatoes. Bring water to a boil.

Reduce heat to medium-low, cover, and let the casserole simmer until water is absorbed and rice is tender, about 20 minutes.

Stir in peas, corn, and beans and cook for 8–10 minutes. When everything is hot, the casserole is ready to serve. Garnish with olives or capers, if desired.

Spanish Omelet
This tasty dish provides a healthy array of vegetables and can be used for breakfast, brunch, or any meal! Serve with fresh fruit salad and a whole grain dinner roll.

Ingredients:
5 small potatoes, peeled and sliced
Vegetable cooking spray
½ medium onion, minced
1 small zucchini, sliced

1½ cups green/red peppers, sliced thin
5 medium mushrooms, sliced
3 whole eggs, beaten
5 egg whites, beaten
Pepper and garlic salt with herbs, to taste
3 ounces shredded part-skim mozzarella cheese
1 Tbsp. low-fat parmesan cheese

Directions:

Preheat oven to 375 °F.

Cook potatoes in boiling water until tender. • In a non-stick pan, add vegetable spray and warm at medium heat.

Add onion and sauté until brown. Add vegetables and sauté until tender but not brown.

In a medium mixing bowl, slightly beat eggs and egg whites, pepper, garlic salt, and low-fat mozzarella cheese. Stir egg-cheese mixture into the cooked vegetables.

In a 10-inch pie pan or ovenproof skillet, add vegetable spray and transfer potatoes and egg mixture to pan. Sprinkle with low-fat parmesan cheese and bake until firm and brown on top, about 20–30 minutes.

Remove omelet from oven, cool for 10 minutes, and cut into five pieces.

Tropical Fruits Fantasia

The tropics offer a great variety of fruits that will make this delicious and colorful recipe stand out; it will also make your mouth water even before tasting it!

Ingredients:
8 ounces fat-free, sugar-free orange yogurt
5 medium strawberries, cut into halves
3 ounces honeydew melon, cut into slices (or ½ cup cut into cubes)
3 ounces cantaloupe melon, cut into slices (or ½ cup cut into cubes)
1 mango, peeled and seeded, cut into cubes
1 papaya, peeled and
seeded, cut into cubes
3 ounces watermelon, seeded and cut into slices (or ½ cup cut into cubes)
2 oranges, seeded and cut into slices
½ cup unsweetened orange juice

Directions:

Add yogurt and all fruits to a bowl and carefully mix together.

Pour orange juice over fruit mixture.

Mix well and serve

Two Cheese Pizza

Serve your pizza with fresh fruit and a mixed green salad garnished with red beans to balance your meal.

Ingredients:
2 Tbsp. whole wheat flour
1 can (10 ounces)refrigerated pizza crust
Vegetable cooking spray
2 Tbsp. olive oil
½ cup low-fat ricotta cheese
½ tsp. dried basil
1 small onion, minced
2 cloves garlic, minced
¼ tsp. salt (optional)
4 ounces shredded part-skim mozzarella cheese
2 cups mushrooms, chopped
1 large red pepper, cut into strips

Directions:

Preheat oven to 425 °F.

Spread whole wheat flour over working surface. Roll out dough with rolling pin to desired crust thickness.

Coat cookie sheet with vegetable cooking spray.

Transfer pizza crust to cookie sheet. Brush olive oil over crust.

Mix low-fat ricotta cheese with dried basil, onion, garlic, and salt. Spread this mixture over crust.

Sprinkle crust with part-skim mozzarella cheese. Top cheese with mushrooms and red pepper.

Bake at 425 °F for 13–15 minutes or until cheese melts and crust is deep golden brown.

Stevia...A Gift From Nature

Stevia is a shrub native to Paraguay and Brazil and has been used by the native Guarani Indians for over 1500 years. The Guarani's used stevia as a natural herbal sweetener to sweeten their bitter drinks such as mate and for medicinal use to treat diabetes and hypertension. It nourishes the pancreas but does not raise normal blood glucose levels, making it safe for diabetics and hypergylcemics. Stevia lowers high blood pressure but does not affect normal blood pressure. Stevia contains an abundance of phytonutrients and trace minerals. The herb also contains no calories or carbohydrates and its antibacterial properties help prevent tooth decay. Stevia is an ideal natural sweetener alternative for sugar and artificial sweeteners such as aspartame. As the herb has no calories or carbohydrates, it acts as a great weight loss aid and digestive aid and helps minimize cravings for sweets, fatty foods and helps with addictions to tobacco and alcohol. Stevia is useful for healing a variety of skin problems. Whole leaf can help soften and tighten the skin and smooth wrinkles. Stevia supreme liquid can be used on acne outbreaks, eczema and lip and mouth sores. Studies show that stevia prevents gum disease and prevents cavities.

Chapter VIII
Managing Diabetes

Exercise for Diabetics

The two most common forms of diabetes are referred to as Type 1 and Type 2. Type 1 diabetes, also known as adolescent diabetes, differs from Type 2 in that the body stops producing insulin altogether. Type 2 diabetes is generally diagnosed in older adults and occurs as the body stops producing enough insulin or the individual becomes resistent to their own insulin.

With either form of diabetes, we lose our ability to adequately untilize sugar. Blood sugar levels increase due to the body's difficulty in transporting sugar into the cells and out of the blood stream. There are various ways to lower blood sugar levels including exercise, diet, and medications.

Exercise is a very important part of diabetic management for both Type 1 and Type 2 diabetics. For the Type 1 diabetic, regular exercise helps to maintain insulin sensitivity, helps prevent accumulation of excess weight, and increases the use of glucose by muscles, thereby lower blood sugar levels. While there is currently no way to prevent Type 1 diabetes, it may be possible to prevent Type 2 diabetes.

Things to consider when attempting to prevent the onset of Type 2 diabetes are regular exercise, supplementation with vitamins and herbs that help prevent insulin resistance, and proper weight control.

Exercise not only helps directly in diabetic management by lowering blood sugar levels and maintaining insulin sensitivity, but also helps minimize many of the complications that can arise in a diabetic individual. Studies have shown that walking for 30 minutes per day can substantially diminish the possibility of developing Type 2 diabetes.

Diabetics tend to develop circulatory problems and exercise can certainly help lower blood pressure and improve circulation throughout the body. Since individuals with diabetes tend to have poor blood flow to their lower extremities and feet, better circulation is of great benefit.

There are some risks associated with exercise, but the potential benefits greatly outweigh the risks. Since exercise does lower blood sugar levels, people with diabetes should measure their blood sugar both before and after exercising. Since your body uses more sugar while exercising and makes you more sensitive to insulin, there is a risk of blood sugar becoming too low and causing hypoglycemia.

When exercising it is important to let others know that you are diabetic. They should be informed what to do in case of hypoglycemia. You should always carry candy or fruit juice to treat low blood sugar levels should they occur. During and after exercise sessions, you should pay close attention to how you feel since rapid heart beat, increased sweating, feeling shaky, or hunger can signal that your blood sugar levels are becoming too low.

Exercise is a critical part of diabetic management and treatment. Exercise helps blood sugar control when the muscles use more glucose and the body become more sensitive to insulin. Exercise also helps to prevent and minimize common diabetic complications including heart problems, high blood pressure and circulatory deficiencies. All diabetics should include a regular exercise program as part of their overall management plan.

Does Alcohol Decreases The Risk Of Diabetes?

Drinking Alcohol Really Does Decreases the Risk of Type 2 Diabetes Among Older Women

It is absurd. For the longest time, we have believed that alcohol has no real benefits. However, recently, a study has found that drinking moderate amounts of alcohol really does decreases the risk of Type 2 Diabetes, and this is especially true among Older Women! There are 20.8 million children and adults in the United States, or 7% of the population, who have diabetes. While an estimated 14.6 million have been diagnosed with diabetes, unfortunately, 6.2 million people (or nearly one-third) are unaware that they have the disease.

Recent studies have shown that drinking moderate amounts of alcohol (as compared to drinking too much alcohol or no alcohol at all) can lower the chances of getting type 2 diabetes. However, only a few studies on alcohol and type 2 diabetes have included women, and very few have included older women.

Previous studies on the effects of drinking moderate amounts of alcohol (1-2 drinks) and the risk of developing type 2 diabetes have mostly been done on men or both men and women who were younger than 55 years old. The researchers wanted to study how drinking alcohol affects older women's (more than 50 years old) chances of developing type 2 diabetes. (see Diabetes Symptoms)

Questionnaires were mailed to the women in the study. The women were asked where they lived and if they had conditions that put them at risk for any other diseases. Waist and hip, height, weight, and blood pressure measurements were taken at the beginning of the study. Diabetes, high blood pressure, and high cholesterol were also reported if these conditions were diagnosed by a doctor. The questionnaire asked about how much each woman exercised and how much they ate.

The questionnaire also contained questions about how much alcohol the women drank, how often they drank, and what types of alcohol they drank, both currently and in the past. The researchers sent out two follow-up questionnaires every 3 to 5 years. These questionnaires asked the women whether they developed type 2 diabetes, what year they were diagnosed, who diagnosed them, and whether they were being treated by diet, drugs, and/or insulin.

Conclusion

The researchers found that blood pressure was lower in the women who drank moderately, but it increased in women who drank more. During the study, a total of 760 new cases of diabetes were diagnosed. The research shows, however, that drinking alcohol in moderate amounts did lessen the risk of developing type 2 diabetes. This is rather significant piece of news as we can now safely drink our favourite wine and not feel guilty about it!

Where To Get Diabetes Supplies

Diabetes has slowly crept into the lives of almost eleven million Americans who have diabetes and are aware they have the illness, and up to seven million Americans who are not aware they have diabetes. Added to this glaring number of diabetes-stricken Americans are the millions more who are in the pre-diabetes stage.

People with diabetes have more chances of surviving the illness if they know how to manage diabetes and they have the financial means to support the medication and other supplies required by people with diabetes.

Getting Type 1 diabetes is usually dependent on you genes although it is not a very strong risk factor. Obesity and age are however risk factors in getting Type 2 diabetes. But no matter how old you are, if you are obese and have a history of gestational diabetes, have one or both parents with Type 2 diabetes or high blood pressure, then it is best to have yourself checked for diabetes.

Type 1 diabetes is commonly found in children while Type 1.5 diabetes is the name given to diabetes found in adults. Adults with Type 1.5 diabetes is characterized by a slower attack on the beta cells compared to the vicious attack of beta cells in children with Type 1 diabetes. In Type 2 diabetes, the body's insulin cannot control its blood sugar levels.

There are several ways of testing for diabetes including the glucose test which measures the blood's glucose level and the oral glucose test. The glucose test is best done after at least 12 hours of fasting.

The main concern for people with diabetes is how to control the level of their blood glucose in such a way that they can lessen diabetes-related complications. Thus, monitoring of one's blood glucose level is always a must for people with diabetes. Controlling the blood glucose level means choosing the type of food you eat and taking the proper medication.

A person who wants to be in control of his diabetes should have all the necessary supplies on hand whether he stays in the house or he travels. A diabetic should always make sure that his insulin supply is not exposed to extreme changes in temperature. A diabetic is also more prone to foot problems so he should take care of his feet by using comfortable socks.

Other important supplies for diabetics include blood glucose monitors, blood pressure monitors, glucose tablets and gels.

If you have diabetes, make sure that you have your supplies wherever you go. Also inform your housemates or officemates about the possible stores where they can buy these supplies in case you have an emergency. Always scout for stores that sell supplies for diabetics near your home or office or where you frequently go. And if you have to travel, make sure you carry more than enough because you never know what might happen. Also check if the places you will go to have some shops which sell the supplies you need.

Avoid fats, meat and meat foods to control diabetes

Fats

The excessive use of fats has been linked to development of diabetes. A recent study at the University of Colorado Health Science Center, USA found that intake of an extra 40g of fat day increases the chances of developing diabetes by three times. Fat rich diet, especially one saturated with animal fat, seems to damage the insulin's effectiveness. Research at the University of Sydney in Australia measured the saturated fatty acids in the muscles cells of older non-diabetic men and the women undergoing surgery and found that higher the presence of saturated fatty acids in the cells, the greater the insulin resistance. On the other hand, higher tissue levels of polyunsaturated fats, particularly fish oil, indicated better insulin activity and lower resistance. Fish oil differs from animal fats in that fish oil contains polyunsaturated fatty acids. One of the fatty acids called omega-3 is especially good for the heart—it lowers cholesterol and protects from atherosclerosis. In fact, the researchers also reported that intake of omega-3 fish oil to the subjects effectively overcame their insulin resistance.

In another study, Jennifer Lovejoy, assistance professor at Louisiana State of University, USA, studied and the eating habits and insulin activity among 45 non-diabetic men and women. About half of them were obese and the remaining half of normal weight. In both cases, higher fat consumption increased insulin resistance. This indicates, says Dr. Lovejoy, that even normal individuals who decrease their insulin efficiency and boost their vulnerability to diabetes.

Meat and Meat Foods

One of the most important nutrition guidelines to follow is to "eat less saturated fat." A quick and simple way to do that is to eliminate meat products. They are high both in saturated fat and cholesterol content. People with diabetes have a greater risk of heart disease earlier in life. The practically useless calories added by saturated fats contribute to above normal body weight and obesity, putting a diabetic at greater of heart disease.

Flesh foods are extremely harmful for diabetes. They increase the toxemic condition underlying the diabetic state and reduce the sugar tolerance. Most diseases of the human body are caused by autointoxication of self-poisoning. The flesh of animals increases the burden on the organs of elimi-nation and overloads and system with animal waste matter and poisons. Chemical analysis has shown that uric acid and other uric poisons contained in the animal body are almost identical to caffeine and nicotine, the poisonous, stimulating principles of coffee, tea and tobacco.

The renowned journal Lancet, reports that a patient of diabetes must be persuaded to consume less animal foods. However, in cold countries where meat and mat products constitute the bulk of the diet, patients of diabetes should limit their intake of animal products to eggs and white meal like fish and poultry. Even their use of should be kept to the minimum; all red meat and red meat products should be eliminated from the diet.

Award Honors Success in Fight Against Diabetes

Ice cream or yogurt? Regular or diet soda? These may not be critical decisions at your dinner table—unless you're one of nearly 18 million Americans living with diabetes today.

People with diabetes face daily challenges. To remain healthy, they must monitor their blood sugar levels, eat a balanced diet and exercise regularly. Some people also need to take insulin to stay alive.

In an effort to recognize champions of these challeng-es, Eli Lilly and Co. established the LillyforLife Achievement Award in 2002. The award celebrates the inspiring achieve-ments of people of all ages who live with diabetes.

Those recognized do not have to be well known or famous for their achievements but can be everyday people who have accomplished or are working toward exceptional personal success.

This year, Lilly has expanded the award program to include not only people with diabetes but also anyone impacted by the condition or involved with the diabetes community.

Categories of submission include: patients age 18 or over; patients age 17 or under; professionals; caretakers or spouses; and journalists.

One person from each category will be selected by a panel of judges to receive this special award. Applicants are eligible to apply for one category. Peer or self-nominations are accepted from the public through Aug. 30, 2004.

Last year, Rick Largent was honored with the first ever LillyforLife Achievement Award. Largent has been living with type 1, or insulin-dependent, diabetes for 25 years. He has faced extraordinary challenges during his life beyond diabetes. An unfortunate accident left him quadriplegic, and he later lost his 19-year-old daughter to cancer.

Largent neglected to control his blood sugar, putting himself at risk for diabetes-related complications. It was not until he began using an insulin pump that he started taking control of his health again.

Largent began traveling cross-country sharing his story and teaching others that anything is possible when diabetes is managed well. He also visited Capitol Hill in an effort to educate policymakers on the dual dilemma of diabetes and disabilities.

Largent's resilience to conquer diabetes and quadriplegia represents the kind of spirit the LillyforLife Achievement Award stands for. As many who live with diabetes know, if the disease is managed, there's no reason you can't achieve your goals.

How To Control Your Diabetes For Life

Here's what researchers know about controlling blood glucose (blood sugar) in people with diabetes: It's not easy, but it can be done. It takes hard work. And it can save your life.

An important new study by the National Institutes of Health (NIH) shows that tight control of blood glucose can reduce the risk of heart attacks and strokes-the number one killer of people with diabetes-by more than half.

For most people with diabetes, keeping blood glucose under tight control isn't easy. The latest data from the Centers for Disease Control and Prevention (CDC) suggest that fewer than 45 percent of Americans with diabetes are reaching the level of control seen in the NIH study. But it can be done, and the National Diabetes Education Program (NDEP) has materials that can help.

The National Diabetes Education Program's Control Your Diabetes. For Life. campaign materials teach people with diabetes how to know their ABCs-what their AIC (a test of blood glucose), Blood pressure, and Cholesterol numbers are, what they should be, and how to work with their health care team to reach those goals. The materials also offer ideas for sticking to a healthy eating plan, ways to stay active with regular physical activity, and other tips for feeling better and staying healthy.

NDEP materials are easy to read, and available in English, Spanish, and in 15 Asian and Pacific Islander languages. They have been tailored for groups at high risk for diabetes, including American Indians and Alaska Natives, African Americans, and Hispanics/Latinos. And all NDEP materials are based on science, backed by the federal government, and copyright free.

For people with diabetes, controlling blood glucose-along with blood pressure and cholesterol-can save their sight, their limbs and their life.

Diabetes Epidemic because of self-inflicted Obesity
Are you eating yourself into diabetes type 2?

Check if you have these 4 eating habits that could contribute to obesity and possibly make you part of the type 2 diabetes epidemic...
One of the greatest contributors to the type 2 diabetes epidemic is reckoned to be obesity brought on by our modern lifestyles.

Are you eating yourself into diabetes type 2?

Check if you have these 4 eating habits that could contribute to obesity and possibly make you part of the type 2 diabetes epidemic...

1) Unconscious eating...No, I don't mean 'sleep-eating' (I wonder if there is such a thing?) I'm talking about automatic eating without any conscious thought to what is happening.

How often do you do something else whilst eating? Watching TV; reading a book; reading a magazine or newspaper; listening to music, a radio show or conversation? If you're anything like me it's probably a rare occasion when you just sit and have a meal, without interruptions.

A recent study carried out by Penn State laboratory showed pre-school children, who consistently watch TV whilst eating, ate up to 33% more than they did when they had a meal without the TV on.

How much extra do you eat, without realizing it, because you are absorbed in a book or TV program?

2) Eating speed.. Ever finished your meal before others? Ever bolted your food down and then felt bloated afterwards?

In a recent Sky TV program Paul McKenna (the famous hypnotherapist) explained how the simple act of slowing down whilst eating; putting your knife and fork down between mouthfuls, can contribute to weight loss.

Think about it, if you're eating more slowly you'll know when you are full. You won't continue eating and get that uncomfortable bloated feeling. And you won't put extra weight on.

Watching that program gave me an 'Aha!' moment, because that's exactly what my father has done all his life. It's a standing joke in the family that he takes so long to eat a meal—he often finishes half-an-hour after everyone else. And guess what? Yep—he's as skinny as a rake. Wish I could say the same about me!

3) Snacking...Are you really hungry when you snack? Or is it that you "just fancy a bite to eat"?

Snacking is probably one of the biggest contributions to weight gain. It's not so much the snacking, it's what you snack on! Cookies /biscuits, chocolate, cakes, snack bars— all these contain massive amounts of sugar that increase the burden on our immune system. If you overload your system with sugar it may not cope, you could end up with insulin resistance and that leads to type 2 diabetes.

Healthy, no added sugar or sugar free snacks are the best options if you MUST snack.

4) Sugary drinks...Do you have a favorite soft drink? If you do, is it a sugar-sweetened drink or a concentrated

sugar-rich fruit juice? And, on a hot day, how much do you drink of that favorite? Half-a-liter? One liter?

It's all added sugar, which not only impacts on your weight, it also impacts on your body's control of the sugar levels in your blood.

In a recent medical study in the US the results indicated that having just one sugar sweetened drink of fruit juice every day made women more susceptible to becoming part of the type 2 diabetes epidemic, by up to 80%.

So, are you planning to be part of the diabetes epidemic? OK, maybe you're not PLANNING to…but maybe your unconscious eating habits have got you on that slippery slope to diabetes. A little thought about what you eat, where and how, can reduce the risk for you.

I have found what I believe the best glucose multi-vitamin herb Blood Sugar Stabilizer By combining Chromium GTF,Vitamin B-12 the trace minerals zinc and vanadium, the major mineral magnesium and the amino acids L-carnitine and L-glutamic acid…..EnZact 77K®, an exclusive enzymatic activation and delivery system, and herbal support from Glucomannan and Gymnema Sylvestre adds further power.

Get Rid of Your Diabetes

Today, there are at least 20 million people living with diabetes in America and the sad part is that it is possible to prevent and heal pre-diabetes and diabetes type 2 naturally with balanced nutrition, and basic exercise.

People at risk of getting the disease drop by a staggering 60 percent if they manage to lose just 10 pounds by following a healthy diet and engage in regular exercise such as walking, according to a report published in the New England Journal of Medicine. (May 3, 2001).

What a product of choice is for CIRCULATORY HEALTH.

Includes herbs like Hawthorne Berry, rhizomes of Butcher's Broom and lipids like CoQ10, EDTA, L-argine and L-carnitine.

Encourage metabolism of fats into metabolites or energy.
Assist with the repair of tissue.
Address blood circulation and stronger capillaries.

A broad-spectrum nutritional supplement that supports cardiovascular health. By providing vital nutrients like vitamins, minerals, amino acids, lipids, herbals, bioflavanoids, enzymes, EDTA and more, and works in harmony with your body to: Counteract free radicals and oxidants that disturb cells, membranes and blood vessels.

Complete the citric acid cycle to complete the energy transfer within the cells.

Selected Benefits:

Assist with the repair of tissue.
Address homocysteine concerns that impact circulatory issues.
Address obstructions.
Activate digestive and tissue healing enzymes.
Address blood circulation and stronger capillaries.
Address blood lipid levels including LDL and HDL cholesterol normal levels.
Encourage metabolism of fats into metabolites or energy.

Together, these ingredients have a time-tested track record for stimulating circulation. That's why it is the foundation of good health.

Calcium

Calcium is the most abundant and the most important mineral in the body, yet it is the most difficult to get absorbed and utilized by the cells.

All degenerative diseases, such as diabetes, cancer, heart disease, gallstones, kidney stones, arthritis, osteoporosis, and many more have been scientifically linked to deficiencies in calcium and other minerals.

Scientists have discovered that the body fluids of healthy people are mildly alkaline (high pH), whereas the body fluids of sick people are acidic (low pH). Calcium is responsible for maintaining the proper body fluid pH.

To stay alive, your blood must remain slightly alkaline. When you drink a cola (highly acidic), take medications or eat foods that are acidic to the body, it uses calcium to buffer the excess acid to keep the pH of the blood slightly alkaline.

If the body can't get the calcium it needs from its reserves, takes it from the bones and this leads to more problems. Thus, calcium reserves are extremely important to maintaining good health

Seaweed Juice

You've heard about the nutritional benefits of kelp— but did you know how difficult it is, thanks to environmental pollution, to find a pure, pristine source? They discovered it in the untouched Pacific paradise of Tonga, the source of superb Limu Moui extract. Then they added advanced Russian adaptogens, the extraordinary performance-enhancing plants uncovered by years of scientific research. According to research, this complex carbohydrate may lend extraordinary support to the body's immune functions. The strength of this does not stop at fucoidan. This revolutionary elixir also contains advanced Russian adaptogens. Adaptogens are a rare class of plant first identified by Russian scientists. In the mid-1950s, the Russian government commissioned its Academy of Sciences to create a product to enhance human performance.

But with modest weight loss and moderate daily physical activity, you can delay or even prevent type 2 diabetes and lead a normal life. Lets look at a few steps you can use straight away in your daily life that will make a big difference to your condition.

Strength Training—Researchers have reported a 23% increase in glucose uptake after four months of strength training. Because poor glucose metabolism is associated with adult onset diabetes, improved glucose metabolism is an important benefit of regular strength exercise.

Nowadays you do not have to live in a gym to put on functional muscle. Short High Intensity sessions performed once a week is all that is required to improve glucose metabolism and lose weight.

The strength training technique I use requires just twenty to thirty mins per week. Gone are the days of the five-day a week program with 6 to 12 sets per body part that, method has never worked. One short intense strength-training workout a week will elevate your metabolism more than you ever thought possible.

The two main components of this technique are the intensity of the exercise and the recovery after the exercise. Infrequent, short, high intensity weight training sessions, followed by the required amount of time to recover and become stronger is what is needed to increase functional lean muscle and improve glucose metabolism.

Nutrition—The way to lose body fat and maintain muscle is to have a food program for life. Quality food and more energy output are the basics you'll need to go for. Bulk foods that fill you up and don't fill you out, foods that are low in fat and sugar which aren't refined should be the ideal.

Small frequent meals should be consumed during the day each containing a little protein to maintain muscle and energy levels. Foods with vital vitamin and mineral supplements should also be taken on a daily basis. A high quality broad-spectrum vitamin and mineral supplement should also be taken on a daily basis.

As before get the calories from high quality food but if you can't, utilize a blender to make concoctions from skim milk with whatever additives you want to use, just as long as you keep count of the calories for your daily total.

Now use these blender mixtures and solid food for your daily feedings. Spread it out over many small meals a day instead of the traditional three meals a day. The way to keep track of weight loss is to buy a calorie counter and record your daily calorie intake for a week.

Exercise—Fat is burned from the body when cells oxidize to release energy in the form of exercise. When the exercise is done slowly to moderately then the majority of energy is taken from the fat stores.

The key to effective aerobic training that burns off maximum fat is long-term consistency not intensity. It doesn't matter if you run a mile, jog a mile or walk a mile you will burn exactly the same amount of calories.

The best exercise by far for the purpose of fat-loss is fast walking either indoors on the treadmill or outdoors. Other aerobic activities are the treadmill, bike, climber or any other training gear found in or out of the Gym.

You can do a lot to lower your chances of getting diabetes. By exercising regularly, reducing fat from your diet and losing weight can all help you reduce the risk of developing type 2 diabetes.

The glycemic index helps us to understand which foods are best and worst for controlling our blood glucose levels.

As we have seen, when blood glucose levels get too high, insulin is released into the bloodstream by the pancreas to help disperse the glucose. The insulin transports the glucose to cells needing extra energy. The cells have "insulin receptors" positioned so that insulin can bind to them, facilitating glucose entry and utilization in the cells. Once inside the cells, the glucose is burned to produce heat and adenosine triphosyphate, (ATP) a molecule that stores and releases energy as required by the cell.

When cells become less sensitive to the effects of insulin, they accept less glucose, so more glucose than usual remains in the bloodstream. Result? The pancreas overcompensates by working harder and releasing even more insulin.

The combination of insulin-insensitivity and insulin over-production typically leads to one of two results:

Either, the pancreas gets worn out and insulin production slows down to abnormally low levels. Result? We develop type 2 diabetes. (About 30 percent of cases)

Or, the insulin-resistant patient doesn't develop diabetes (because the pancreas continues to produce sufficient insulin) but, instead, contracts hyperinsulinism (abnormally high levels of insulin in the blood), which can cause chronic obesity as well as high blood pressure, high levels of triglycerides, low HDL (good) cholesterol, heart disease, and possibly some cancers.

Appetizer Diet Cookies and Protien Shakes

What I have found to be the easiest way to eat fast.. is the diet cookie and protein shakes, these are also perfect for controlling your blood sugar, and are inexpensive. A meal replacement costs about $3.00 breakfast and lunch... so when you realize you don't have to buy food for breakfast or lunch.. it really doesn't cost anything because you have to eat,... and any food will cost you that. One thing to keep in mind about this is sometimes when I eat the cookie (it has a lot of fiber) I really don't want the shake but I force myself to drink it. I've tried not drinking it and every time I don't drink it later on…. usuallyin the evenings I start craving food… usually the wrong kind…. So I just make a point to take the shake whether I feel like or not. It just gives your body the proper nutrients so it doesn't crave food

Support Of Diabetes From The Family

Not to be missed in the treatment of diabetes is support from the people we love. In truth, one reference notes that "the quality of a family's time can be mutually beneficial" in managing diabetes in the family with juveniles or adults.

It is beneficial when those in the family are trained about diabetes. Knowledge will lend a hand of support to the diabetic. You'll recognize imperative symptoms, and know how to take action. One family who offers support to their diabetic relatives noted how they can recognize changes in each other when medical treatment is needed.

Being able to detect symptoms like being sweaty, shaky or impatient will help caring family members to take charge of any diabetic situations.

Loving family members must strive to be supportive and patient with their diabetic family members. This support can be invaluable coming from within the family for the diabetic. The greatest support group is at home with love and care. Family and friends in addition want to understand that as blood-sugar levels fluctuate, diabetes can affect one's moods.

A family member would never want to belittle or make fun of a spouse, sibling, daughter or son because of diabetes. Too, remembering that they have limitations on what they eat we may also follow their same diet plan. Never would we want to tempt them to eat something that could make them sick.

Remember you are an important part of your diabetic relatives successful treatment. They may not show it but you mean a lot to them. If you just give them some words of encouragement like they are doing great what a world of difference that will mean to them. Treat them like normal people with circumstances to care for.

Diabetes can be managed effectively, specially if the sufferer has cooperation from friends and family.

Chapter IX
Weight Loss

Affirming Habits

Have you ever caught yourself trying to get rid of negative habits by forcefully resisting them? For example, when you find yourself tempted by actions that do not support your weight loss goals, do you get angry and try to "shout" the cravings down? Mentally you say, "No! I will not eat that cookie. I don't need it and it's not on my food plan. I refuse to be a weakling about food or anything else." Though common, this type of negative reinforcement is rarely effective, simply because it moves you into a negative state of mind and it's hard to make positive choices from a negative state of mind.

What you could do instead, however, is begin consciously affirming the positive habits that you are trying to adopt. For example, when you begin your daily workout say to yourself with feeling, "I really love the way working out makes me feel. I'm getting stronger and stronger every day, and soon my workouts will get much easier." As you prepare a healthful meal for yourself say, "This food looks so delicious. I love nourishing my body with foods that are bursting with vitamins and goodness."

And what should you do with the negative habits? Give them as little attention as possible. Simply switch your focus away from temptations and don't make a big deal out of them. Remember, the more attention and focus you give them, the more power you give them.

Do the same thing if you have an off day and make a few unhealthy decisions. Rather than obsessing about the slip and beating yourself up over it, simply admit that you made some bad decisions and vow to do better beginning now. Pat yourself on the back for continuing to try improving your habits, and affirm that you will keep getting better. Over time as you continue to reinforce your positive habits and minimize your focus on the negative habits, you'll find that you naturally gravitate toward the positive.

Being Lightness

In this day and age we are learning more and more about the power of our thoughts and the way they contribute heavily to our perceptions on a physical level. Have you ever felt like you made something happen by thinking obsessively about it? I'm not talking about magical powers here, but rather your own perception of your experiences and the outer events that seem to correspond with them.

For example, have you ever gotten dressed up for an event that you really didn't want to attend and didn't have any clothes you felt comfortable wearing? You probably felt uncomfortable through the whole event, worried that other people were talking about you behind your back, and in fact you may have even seen people whispering while looking in your direction. Maybe they were talking about you and maybe they weren't—but the important thing is that you believed they were.

Just like a negative focus can contribute to negative experiences, it is also possible to use this same concept to feel better about yourself. One way to do this is by performing a "lightness" meditation every day. If you begin to focus more of your attention on feeling light, slender and beautiful, you just might begin to have more experiences that correspond with such a mind-set!

Here's how to do a Lightness meditation. Once or twice a day, find a place where you can lie down and not be disturbed for 10 or 15 minutes. Take a few slow, deep breaths and focus on quieting your body and mind. Then, imagine that you begin to feel a warm, soothing humming sensation flowing over you, relaxing away all tension. Imagine that your body begins to feel lighter, and the pressure of your body against the bed or sofa begins to lessen. Feel yourself getting slimmer and lighter with each moment that passes, until it feels like you are actually floating a few inches above the surface you are lying on. When you come out of this meditation, you should definitely feel lighter, slimmer and better about your body—and it gets more powerful each time you do it.

Believing in a New You

Your beliefs have a lot more to do with your lifestyle than you may think; everything from your body size to your level of fitness to the types of food you eat most often—and more. Basically, everything you do or don't do in life is based on a set of beliefs that support the actions. For example, you may have always avoided exercise because you kept telling yourself you didn't like it. Or you may have told yourself since childhood that you don't enjoy eating vegetables.

Questioning and examining these beliefs is important because you may find that they have been holding you back from achieving your health goals. Spend time each day exploring your beliefs about yourself, your body, your health, and everything else related to your current goals. Write down what you believe to be true about these things. Your list might look something like this: "It's hard for me to lose weight because I have a slow metabolism. I never lose weight on low fat diets, only low carb. I inherited my mother's genes; she's overweight just like me." As you write these things down, think carefully about them and consider whether they are really true or not. You may be surprised to discover that some of these beliefs are misleading or downright false.

Once you identify a false or otherwise limiting belief, begin changing it by telling yourself a new story. After all, that's exactly what your existing beliefs are—stories you have been telling yourself for years! Your new story might go something like this: "It's true that my metabolism has slowed down some over the years, but I can boost it again by eating healthful foods and working out each day. I will lose weight naturally just by moderating my intake of carbs and fat. I may have inherited the tendency for obesity from my mother, but I can still choose to live a healthy or unhealthy lifestyle and my body weight will be affected either positively or negatively because of it."

As you change the stories you tell yourself, you change your own behaviors and ultimately, your results!

Carry With Confidence

Increased confidence is undoubtedly a great benefit of losing weight. When you're fit and healthy you just feel better about yourself, and that confidence gets carried into every aspect of your life. You're better at your work, your relationships tend to deepen and become richer, and even your day to day activities seem to take on a more positive hue. The problem is that most of us tend to equate this increased confidence with the finality of that last excess pound dropping off, when it really doesn't have anything to do with the weight loss itself.

Rather than looking forward to the day when you finish losing weight because you think it will make you feel more confident, why not begin working on boosting your confidence now?

Here are two easy ways to do it:

- Feel good about yourself now.

You may think that having a slim body is what makes you feel good about yourself, but it's actually your own thoughts! As the weight drops off, you inevitably begin thinking more positively about yourself; thoughts like, "I'm really proud of myself; I'm doing so well; I feel really good; I know I'm going to reach my goals; I'm looking great..." and so on. Start thinking those thoughts now, and you'll find yourself feeling more confident even before you've lost your first pound.

- Take pride in your appearance.

Most people dream of wearing beautiful clothes after they are thin, but settle for looking frumpy and disheveled while they are still losing weight. While you may not want to invest in a new wardrobe for every size along the way to your goal, you can still make an effort to wear clothing that makes you feel good now. Get rid of clothes that are much too big or old and faded. Take care to be well-groomed in other ways too, like your hair, and do what you can to be presentable in every way you can. Take pride in your appearance and you won't be able to help feeling more confident.

Cathartic Creativity

When you're trying to change your lifestyle habits and make healthier choices, you may find yourself dealing with a lot of stress and anxiety that you're not sure how to handle.

This is especially true if you have gotten into the habit of using food as a cover for negative emotions.

One healthy way to process your feelings is by engaging in creative pursuits. There's something so satisfying about channeling stress, anxiety and anger through activities that leave you feeling clear, refreshed and fully connected to your authentic self. If you've never tried this, you'll want to start by coming up with a list of creative activities that you enjoy so you can quickly turn to them when you find yourself feeling unsettled. If you currently have no hobbies, think back to your childhood and young adult years. What kind of activities did you enjoy most? What type of creative classes did you take in school? Write them down.

Also take some time to think about activities you haven't yet explored but want to. Have you always been fascinated by dance or theater? Do you love browsing through floral shops and gazing at the beautiful arrangements? Make a list of your interests, as well as ideas for activities you can do to pursue them. Begin buying the supplies you'll need for these activities gradually. If budget is a concern, perhaps you can trade supplies with a friend or start on a smaller scale with just one type of creative activity for now.

Finally, begin engaging in these activities as often as you can, and especially when you feel troublesome emotions beginning to creep in. Sing out your sorrow. Write dark poetry to express your anger. Paint beautiful scenes to express your love of life. Yes, you can do this for positive emotions too, not just negative. Over time, you will get used to naturally expressing your feelings without turning to food, and eating and living consciously will become a habit all its own.

YOGA

Many times, people embark on a wellness journey which includes yoga training There are many different "styles" of yoga, just as there are many different yoga teachers and "styles" of teaching. It is important that each person realize their personal yoga practice is just that – personal – and although there may be other students in a class, each class is a personal and different experience for each student. You make your yoga journey unique by focusing on yourself, your body, your challenges, your capabilities, and your current state of mind during that particular hour. Give yourself that gift.

There are many different styles of yoga being taught and practiced today. Although all of the styles are based on the same physical postures (called poses or asanas), each has a particular emphasis.

Hatha is a very general term that can describe different types of yoga. If a class is described as Hatha style, it is typically a slow-paced and gentle and provides a good introduction to basic yoga poses.

Anusara combines a strong emphasis on physical alignment with a positive philosophy derived from Tantra. The philosophy's premise is belief in the intrinsic goodness of all beings. Anusara classes are usually light-hearted and accessible to students of differing abilities. Poses are taught in a way that opens the heart, both physically and mentally, and props are often used. This is considered a gentle yoga

Vinyasa, which means breath-synchronized movement, tends to be a more vigorous style based on the performance of a series of poses called Sun Salutations, in which movement is matched to the breath. If you have never tried yoga you will be amazed at the results.

Avoiding painful or uncomfortable feelings is one of the most common destructive habits that many people struggle with, and more often than not food or other substances are used to numb or cover the feelings that they don't know how to deal with in healthy ways. Needless to say, this type of habit can wreak havoc on your weight loss goals. You can avoid this happening to you if you learn how to get and stay in touch with your feelings and come up with positive ways to comfort yourself when life gets difficult.

First and foremost, it is necessary to begin paying attention to the way you feel throughout the day. Get into the habit of tuning in mentally to your emotional state. Ask yourself questions like, "How do I feel right now? Am I happy or sad? Angry or peaceful?" If you notice that you are struggling with negative emotions, do a little digging to figure out why. Ask yourself, "What made me feel angry? Why do I feel sad right now?"

Then, do your best to process and release the feelings. You may not be able to resolve all of the root causes for these feelings right away, but often just knowing why you feel the way you do is enough. Then commit to working through the feelings rather than being tempted to cover them up or run away again.

At the same time, get into the habit of doing things that comfort you on a regular basis. You don't have to spend a lot of time on these activities, but do at least one or two small things for yourself each day, like taking a relaxing bubble bath, going for an invigorating walk, meditating, journaling, taking short cat naps when you feel tired, or anything else you enjoy doing. Even just a few minutes of nurturing and comforting yourself can go a long way in easing emotional turbulence—and you'll find that you don't need to overeat to do it.

Core of Worth

When you think of losing weight, you probably equate it to moving from a "bad" state (fat) to a "good" state (thin). You may view your extra pounds as evil, disgusting creatures that have no right occupying space on your body, and you may even feel a bit disgusted with yourself for gaining the pounds in the first place. This is a common feeling, but it can be incredibly damaging and continue to perpetuate the cycle of "bad and good"—even once you have lost weight.

In order to achieve truly lasting, healthy weight loss, you need to be thinking and acting from a core of worth.

Your core of worth is the foundation of belief that you truly deserve to be healthy, strong and happy. Do you currently have such a foundation? Or do you think about yourself and your weight along the lines of good or bad? You may think that punishing yourself into losing weight by thinking of your fat (and yourself) as being gross and out of control will be effective, but it actually creates more resistance within you.

As a result, you continue to feel badly about yourself, treat your body poorly and eat more than you should. If you then try to use that same mind-set to lose the excess weight, you will only make yourself feel worse and find it harder and harder to lose weight.

To achieve a healthy body and mind, you need to begin loving and believing in yourself. You need to believe that you deserve to be healthy and happy, and let your actions flow naturally from that belief. You need to act from a core of worth that says, "I deserve better than what I've been givng myself up to now." When you approach weight loss with this type of attitude, treating yourself kindly becomes much easier. Keep saying to yourself every day, "I deserve to be treated kindly. I deserve to eat foods I love and that make my body feel good". When you do this, your whole life becomes much more balanced and you don't have to fight those inner and outer "demons" that kept you tied to unhealthy habits for so long.

becomes much more balanced and you don't have to fight those inner and outer "demons" that kept you tied to unhealthy habits for so long.

Encouraging Words

Have you ever become aware of your own self-talk? Each of us has a constant stream of self-talk flowing through our mind at any given moment, but most often it is on a subconscious level so we're not aware of it. Unfortunately, you may be in the same boat as many other people, with the majority of your self-talk being negative or derogatory. Without even realizing it you may be constantly telling yourself how stupid you are, how fat you are, you'll never succeed at anything, and so on.

The good news is that even though you may not be aware of your self-talk much of the time, you can still take control of it by choosing to speak more positively to yourself on a regular basis. This will eventually override those old negative messages that have been playing in your head for years. The way to do this is simple: begin talking to yourself with positive words and in a positive tone as often as you can. You can wake up and say, "I really feel good about myself today," or "I'm a great person and I love myself." When you do something well, congratulate yourself. When you screw up, comfort yourself and affirm that it's okay. The idea is to become a source of love and encouragement for yourself, rather than abuse and ridicule.

You can also do this in written form, which is sometimes even more effective than spoken words. Spend a few minutes every morning and/or evening writing a nice letter to yourself. You can write general nice things like, "You are such a good person; you are very compassionate and kind, and you always try hard to listen when people talk to you". Or you can get more specific like, "I really admire the way you handled the pressure at work today". It doesn't matter what you choose to focus on, just that you are building yourself up and transmitting positive messages to yourself.

Whether you do it verbally or in written form, get into the habit of encouraging and building yourself up. Think, speak and act kindly toward yourself, and you will find yourself transforming from powerless victim to empowered, confident person in record time.

Expecting Success

With almost every weight loss attempt, there is an underlying sense of "walking on eggshells". Have you ever felt like you must do everything exactly right or be doomed to failure? Have you ever worried that "this time" would end up being like all the rest of the times you've tried to lose weight and couldn't stick to it?

This line of thought stems from fear and it is more destructive than you can imagine. Why? Because the more you fear or worry about something, you are more likely to act in ways that perpetuate it. For example, if you fear that one wrong move will ruin your diet completely, what do you think will happen if you do slip up and eat a food that is not on your plan? Most likely you'll conclude that you have failed and throw in the towel. Underlying this fear of failure is the belief that you will fail no matter how hard you try to succeed.

Don't allow fear-based thinking to destroy your attempts to create a better life. Begin today by expecting success with your healthy habits and everything else you want in life. Learn to see minor slip-ups as learning experiences. Analyze them and understand why they happened, and come up with ways to prevent them from happening again. Develop a better awareness of your own strengths and weaknesses, and strive to improve in all areas—not from an unrealistic expectation of perfection, but from a desire to do the very best you can in everything you do.

Start each day with a positive expectation of success. Believe you are already successful, and you are becoming more successful every day. Just like fearing failure makes it more likely to happen, expecting success make it much more likely to happen. You just have to choose which one you will give most of your focus to.

Feeding Your Soul

Have you ever caught yourself eating when you weren't hungry or craving specific foods for no apparent reason? More often than not, cravings like this come from a deeper place—and you're not craving food at all. You might instead be craving love, comfort, rest, pleasure, or any other number of emotional qualities. Why do these cravings get translated into food cravings? Because many of us have formed a habit of using food and other substances to avoid facing our emotional needs.

Not surprisingly, habits like these can be deeply ingrained, or even completely subconscious. We don't know that our craving for a deluxe bacon cheeseburger is really a desire to be loved and comforted. We just know we want the burger and we want it right now! If we can't have it, we feel miserable.

Introspection and awareness can help you learn to decipher these cravings and figure out what you truly need. One good way to do this is through journaling questions and answers. When a random craving comes over you, grab a sheet of paper and write, "I'm having a craving for _____. Why do I want this?" Then write down the answers that come to mind first. Your answers will vary, but you may first find yourself replying, "Because it will taste good. Because I'm hungry for something besides salad. Because I deserve to eat foods I love."

As you continue to ask more probing questions and dig a little deeper, you'll usually get to the heart of the matter. Then you might start getting answers like, "Because I'm sick of always doing everything for everyone else and not taking care of myself." Do you see the true need within that statement? An answer like this means you are truly craving a little self-care and nurturing! And you can get that in many ways, not by eating a cheeseburger. Once you have identified your true need, you may still have to employ a bit of willpower to do what you know is right because you may still have an irrational emotional attachment to eating a cheeseburger. But the more you get into the habit of feeding your soul, the less of these random cravings you'll experience on a regular basis.

Fit Focus

Have you ever worked out while your thoughts were drifting off in the distance somewhere? Maybe you spend your workouts dreaming about the new wardrobe you're going to buy, brainstorming new business strategies, or fantasizing about your favorite celebrity. But did you know that this habit can reduce the effectiveness of your workouts? Like anything else in life, paying partial attention and giving partial effort usually yields diluted results.

If you want to boost the results you get from exercise, start giving it your full focus while you work out. Focus in on each muscle group as you work it, and concentrate on getting your form just right. Feel your heart and lungs working and the blood flowing through your veins. Breathe deeply and invest yourself mentally and emotionally into the act of flexing and working your body.

Why would you want to do this? Because when you give your full focus to something, you invest a lot more effort into it! Think about the last activity that you were fully immersed in. Maybe you completed a project for school or work, or accomplished a personal goal. Didn't time seem to fly by while you were focused so intently? And didn't the actions you took seem more enjoyable?

When you give your full attention to working out, you will notice a big difference in the way you feel after a work-out—and you will definitely notice better results in your body. You may even begin to really enjoy your workouts because for the first time you are fully present while doing them—rather than trying desperately to escape them mentally. If you've never allowed yourself to engage fully with your activities like this before, try it and see what a difference it can make in both your attitude and your physical conditioning.

Honor the Temple

You've probably heard it said that the body is a temple for the spirit, but how often do you act in ways that truly honor and respect your body? Forget all the religious connotations and think about a temple as a "holy place"—or a place of sacred connection. Would you ever enter a holy place and throw garbage around? Would you verbally abuse the residents living there? Would you paint obscene graffiti on the walls? Most of us are horrified by the thought—but we think nothing of treating our own "temple" with such disregard.

You may be thinking, "I don't treat myself that badly," and maybe you don't. But can you honestly say that you treat your body with reverence and love? If you are like most people, you have not been taught how to do that. Most of us were taught the exact opposite; that we should always put others before ourselves. Selflessness may have its merits, but it's also important to value and love yourself.

One of the easiest ways to begin honoring yourself is by treating yourself the same way you would treat someone you loved dearly. From this moment on, vow to treat yourself as if you were the person you loved most in the world. Treat yourself as if you were someone very special, someone who should always be revered and honored no matter what—just like a holy temple is.

Make decisions that support your mental, physical, emotional and spiritual wellness. Approach your healthy lifestyle with joy and love, not rigidity and force. When you begin seeing your body as a holy place, you will find that you have a much harder time treating it carelessly. You automatically want to care for it properly, and you naturally take the steps to do so.

Patient Progress

It can often seem to take forever to see results. You wish you could fast-forward your life to the day when you are already thin so you don't have to go through the grueling process of losing all those pounds between now and then. In fact, some people may even take drastic measures to speed up the process by severely restricting caloric intake or engaging in even more destructive behaviors. When this happens, it is usually because the person is so desperate to reach the "Thin" finish line that they sacrifice their own health for the sake of being thin.

Hopefully you see the benefits of following a healthy, balanced program to lose weight gradually, but you may still feel impatient that your weight loss is taking too long. In order to make the waiting easier, you may want to devise some mental strategies to keep you feeling satisfied that progress is being made, rather than getting frustrated that you're not moving fast enough.

One of the best ways to do this is by consistently looking back and confirming how far you've come. Even if you haven't experienced massive results yet, you can still acknowledge the inner and outer changes taking place and affirm that more are in progress. You can take a few "before" and "during" photos to help keep yourself inspired, or even keep a running log of your weight and body measurements so you can see clearly that you are making progress. When you do this, you shift from feeling stuck to knowing that you are always moving forward, and that alone can be satisfying enough until the bigger results start showing.

More often than not, every phase of a weight loss journey is directly related to your own attitude. If you feel like you aren't moving fast enough, if you are overly dependent upon getting the end result you want, you will make yourself miserable through the entire journey. But if you can step back and find a way to enjoy where you are now, feel good about how far you've come and look forward to the next phase without being too attached to it, you will strike the perfect balance to make your journey swift and rewarding.

The Time is Now

Keep focusing on the future, looking forward to that glorious day when you are thin. Most often this is because you believe that everything in your life will be good when you are thin. You pin all of your hopes for happiness and contentment to the experience of being thin—but being thin won't make you happy. True, you may feel better both physically and mentally, have more energy and confidence, and you may even be more outgoing and do things you would hesitate to attempt while heavy.

It's a good thing to look forward to future successes, but it's not so good to focus obsessively on them. Why? Because it keeps you forever disconnected from this moment in time. That becomes a problem because you start putting your life off until you reach your goal, which just keeps you in a state of limbo. And you will never reach your goals by keeping yourself in limbo!

If you want to speed up your transformation, start being the thin version of yourself NOW. Start thinking, speaking and acting as a person who is confident and slender. Here's an easy way to begin doing this. Make a list of everything you are looking forward to experiencing when you reach your goal. For example, "Feeling good about myself. Being more confident. Having more energy. Wearing nicer clothes." And then come up with ways to begin doing these things now.

Start making an effort to feel good about yourself right now. Be more confident right now. Imagine that you have more energy right now. Wear clothes that make you feel good now. Granted, this takes a bit of imagination because you'll probably feel like you are lying to yourself or putting on an act. And in some ways you will be. But the more you do it, the easier it will get and before you know it, you really WILL be living these things, rather than continuously gazing off into the future, hoping and waiting for your dream life to arrive.

Trusting the Process

Every person who has ever followed a weight loss program has undoubtedly encountered the same frustrating experience: the dreaded plateau. You can be going along just great, sticking to your eating plan, working out on schedule, doing everything you know will help you reach your goal in record time—and then suddenly the results stop coming. The scale gets stuck and you can't seem to make it move downward again no matter what you do. This phenomenon can last anywhere from a day to weeks on end.

Many people when encountering this situation automatically think they must be doing something wrong. They look back over their food journal for clues about what might be stopping their weight loss, they worry that maybe they have a medical condition that will prevent them from losing any more weight, or worse—they simply conclude they have failed and give up.

As frustrating and perplexing as plateaus can be, more often than not they occur for a good reason. Sometimes your body just needs to stay where it is and adjust to the changes you are making. Sometimes you may indeed need to make some minor tweaks to your program in order to nudge the scale downward again. But one thing you should never do is get angry at your body.

Instead, your weight loss journey will be much easier if you learn to see plateaus as just another part of the process of getting to a healthy, fit state of being. It doesn't mean you are doing anything wrong or your body is punishing you. It doesn't mean you are a failure and will always be fat. It just means that you need to be patient and trust the process. Do what you can to determine whether you can improve in certain areas but at the same time, trust the process. Trust your body's wisdom. The scale WILL continue to move if you don't panic and do something drastic. Simply take it one step at a time, and you'll get where you want to be.

Soaring the Heart

One negative aspect of many weight loss programs is that they focus heavily on the "negatives". Don't eat this, you can't have that, you must do this even if you don't want to, and so on. While the actions themselves may be necessary, it is not always necessary to approach everything with such a serious and foreboding attitude. Doing so virtually guarantees that you won't enjoy the journey to your goal weight—you'll simply grit your teeth and bear it, knowing that there is a payoff somewhere down the road.

But it doesn't have to be so dreary! Instead, you can make your weight loss journey much more pleasant—even uplifting—if you make a commitment to doing one thing each day: soaring your heart. What does that mean? It means doing things that make you feel wonderful. Don't dismiss the idea too quickly—it has been proven time and again that your state of mind in anything you do usually determines the quality of results you get. Go into something with a negative mind-set, get lackluster results. Go into it with a positive and optimistic attitude, get great results.

How can this process be applied to your weight loss program? There are a couple of different ways. First, it's important to spend time each day making yourself feel good. You can read inspiring books and magazines, watch uplifting films or television shows, or even join a local support group of likeminded people. Make it your main objective each day to do something that lifts your heart and makes you feel great.

Beyond that, you will also want to apply this same attitude to everything related to your weight loss program. Rather than complaining about the food plan or groaning about your exercise program, enjoy them! Find ways to make everything you do fun and inspiring. Write positive notes to yourself and stick them on your refrigerator and water bottle. Sing while you're working out. Do whatever you can to make the whole process pleasant in some way, and you will find yourself actually enjoying every step on your journey to a better, healthier you

Listening to Inner Wisdom

Living a truly healthy lifestyle involves much more than eating less—it requires learning to listen to your inner wisdom and make choices based on it.

You may not realize it, but your body has its own natural wisdom regarding food and beverage choices, and even the type of physical activities that make it feel best. This wisdom usually communicates with you through bodily sensations and subtle signals. Have you ever gotten an upset stomach after eating one of your favorite foods? Have you ever felt extremely sluggish after eating a big meal? Have you ever forced yourself to eat foods that don't seem to sit well with your body? All of these situations are great examples of not listening to your body's inner wisdom.

Tapping into this inner wisdom is as simple as learning to pay attention and listen. This can be challenging to do because you may be used to making decisions according to habit or cultural conditioning, but it's a process that is well worth learning because it will result in a much more balanced way of living. Here's how to start: first, begin developing a keen awareness of how your body feels moment to moment each day. Periodically, mentally "tune in" and pay attention to how you feel all over. Does your stomach feel okay? Do you have enough energy? Are you thirsty or hungry? Use this checking-in process especially when you eat, drink or engage in physical activities. How does it make your body feel?

Over time, you'll begin to notice that your body sends you very clear signals when you do something that doesn't agree with it. You may get indigestion after eating something heavy, or you may feel tired after a too-intense workout. This doesn't mean you can't make changes, because it's true that even positive changes may feel a bit uncomfortable at first. But at least by listening to your body's wisdom, you will move more comfortably toward better health, rather than trying to force it.

When to Say When

Most of us have completely lost touch with our body's natural trigger for satiety. We may begin eating a meal to address our physical hunger, but continue eating long after our stomach is satisfied—purely for emotional reasons. Can you tell when your body has had enough food? Or is an empty plate your signal to stop eating?

One of the easiest ways to control your food intake is to simply pay attention to when your body says, "enough". Believe it or not, your body does let you know when it has received enough food for the present moment. The problem occurs when you stop listening. For example, have you ever been out at a restaurant enjoying a great meal with friends, when suddenly you realize that you are stuffed to the gills? Fullness hits you like a ton of bricks, and suddenly you realize you have moved beyond "full" into "extremely uncomfortable". You may have heard it said that it takes 20 minutes for your stomach to send a signal to your brain that you are full, but if you pay close attention to your body while eating you'll realize that there are subtle clues that take place even before that happens.

First you will notice after several bites that you no longer feel those empty stomach symptoms, like rumbling, growling, and hollowness. Next you'll probably notice that you feel good—not necessarily full but definitely more satisfied. Finally you'll feel a subtle "click"; an inner shift where you just know that your body is saying, "Good, I've had enough to eat."

Of course, in order to recognize these signals, you need to be paying attention. That means avoiding being distracted while eating and focusing as much of your attention on your meal as you can. This is not always easy to do, but it's necessary if you want to learn to eat more consciously. Remember too that conscious eating takes practice, especially if you have gotten out of touch with your own body. The more you make an effort to stay connected and aware, the better you'll be able to discern your body's signals and know when to say "when".

Take any kind of action if you are diabetic just following what you doctor tells you.. The optional methods of exercise, proper diet, supplementing with real food nutrients and enzymes is a key factor in keeping your body as healthy as possible.

It's virtually impossible to get all the nutrition you need from today's food supply. Our farm soil is depleted of minerals and most of our food supply highly processed. What I have now discovered, has made my disease turn in the other direction instead of continuing to get worse. My body is getting the proper nutrition to heal itself and has restored my energy levels. My Endocrinologist agrees, I'm on the right track. My agenda is to share what I learn with as many people with type II, who are interested in finding alternate ways to help them with stopping the progression.